THE SOUTH BEACH DIET Cookbook

Dr ARTHUR AGATSTON

AUTHOR OF *THE SOUTH BEACH DIET*

RODALE

This edition first published in the UK in 2004 by
Rodale International Ltd
7–10 Chandos Street
London W1G 9AD
www.rodale.co.uk

Recipes on pages 31, 36, 39, 42, 45, 46, 48, 49, 50, 54, 58, 61, 63, 66, 68, 74 (top), 77, 78, 84, 89, 94, 96, 101, 104, 107, 117, 121, 124, 126, 127, 130, 132, 134, 142, 143, 144, 145, 146, 148, 149, 150, 151, 152, 168, 178, 179, 187, 189, 193, 196, 200, 202, 203, 212, 215, 223, 224, 228, 240, 246, 247, 249, 250, 251, 255, 258, 262, 278, 286, 293, 294, 298, 301, 302, 304, 316, 317, 318, 321, 322, 325 remain © Rodale Inc.

Photographs © 2004 Rodale Inc.

Printed in China
Printed on paper from sustainable sources

1 3 5 7 9 8 6 4 2

Jacket and book design by Carol Angstadt
Food styled by Diane Vezza
Props by Melissa DeMayo
Photographs by Mitch Mandel

A CIP record for this book is available from the British Library
ISBN 1–4050–6717–9

Distributed to the book trade by Pan Macmillan Ltd

Notice

This book is intended as a reference volume only, not as a medical manual. The information given here is designed to help you make informed decisions about your health. It is not intended as a substitute for any treatment that may have been prescribed by your doctor. If you suspect that you have a medical problem, we urge you to seek competent medical help.

Mention of specific companies, organizations, or authorities in this book does not imply endorsement by the publisher, nor does mention of specific companies, organizations, or authorities imply that they endorse this book.

Internet addresses given in this book were accurate at the time it went to press.

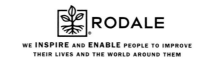

RODALE
WE **INSPIRE** AND **ENABLE** PEOPLE TO IMPROVE
THEIR LIVES AND THE WORLD AROUND THEM

For my sons, Evan and Adam, who have always been interested and enthusiastic supporters of my work. My wish is that you, too, find passion and satisfaction in your chosen professions.

And, as always, to my wife and partner, Sari, for her counsel, her support, and her love.

ACKNOWLEDGEMENTS

First and foremost, I'd like to thank my patients and followers of *The South Beach Diet*. You helped make the first book a tremendous success, and your ideas and feedback have been invaluable. In addition, your strong support has helped promote discussion about healthy eating that is so important.

A very special thank you to my wife, Sari, who worked long and hard on the creation of this book and to Marie Almon, our nutritionist, for her tremendous help developing recipes and overseeing the nutritional aspect of the project.

My editor, Margot Schupf, has been a real partner in this effort and a delight to work with. Jennifer Reich, Carol Angstadt, Mitch Mandel and Diane Vezza were especially instrumental on the design and production side of things. I would also like to acknowledge and thank the entire team at Rodale, including Tami Booth, Amy Rhodes, Cindy Ratzlaff and Cathy Gruhn. Another note of thanks to Lee Brian Schrager and Terry Zarikian for their help in bringing the great chefs of South Beach to this project.

And finally, thanks to Heidi Krupp, my publicist, for her tremendous enthusiasm, and to Richard Pine, my literary agent, for his sound advice and friendship.

CONTENTS

INTRODUCTION

The South Beach Diet was made for people who love to eat.

That will be obvious to anyone who pays attention to current trends in cooking and eating. But you don't have to be a gourmet chef to know what I'm talking about – it's evident in every restaurant menu, every magazine and newspaper article, every television cookery show about how we eat now. Today's best cuisines make use of a wide variety of fresh, wholesome, delicious foods prepared in exciting yet healthy ways.

Similarly, the South Beach Diet encourages you to eat a great variety of foods and to cook them in a healthy manner. On this diet, you can have abundant quantities of nearly any kind of meat or fish you can name. Vegetables and fruit, too. And because the South Beach programme is neither low-carb nor low-fat, you'll be enjoying many of the dishes that other diets require you to give up completely. On our plan, you will eat meals that fully satisfy your hunger; you are even urged to have between-meal snacks and desserts. The types of recipes we offer in this book could be found in any popular cookbook.

Another reason why I say this diet is for food lovers is because of one of its main principles: that we've become an overweight society because we eat too many processed foods. These contain the 'bad' carbohydrates – such as white flour and white sugar – where much of the digestion has begun in factories instead of in our stomachs. This causes our bodies to store excess fat, especially around our middles. Eating these bad carbs also creates cravings for more unhealthy foods; instead of simply satisfying our hunger, they actually make it worse. Eating fewer processed carbohydrates and more dishes made from good, wholesome ingredients will almost automatically bring about weight loss and improved overall health. You'll eat well, too – maybe better than you have in a long time. That's another good reason for a South Beach cookbook. I hope that once you've tried some of the recipes, you'll agree.

As I write this, *The South Beach Diet*, based on the eating plan I developed, is atop the bestseller lists. Later in this book, I will explain the diet itself and how it came to exist. For now, suffice it to say that the programme grew out of my concerns as a cardiologist for the health and well-being of my patients.

If you're already familiar with the South Beach Diet, you'll know that the diet is divided into three phases. To help make things easy for you, every recipe in this book is marked to indicate a phase of the diet – recipes marked as Phase 1 can be enjoyed from the very beginning. Recipes marked as Phase 2 can be enjoyed after you've reached that point in the diet. And Phase 3 recipes are for when you've fully integrated the diet into your lifestyle. There are also 25 recipes from prominent chefs that will make your mouth water. And they all fit into the diet!

Another feature of this book is the shopping list beginning on page 13. This will help you decide what to buy at the supermarket, what to look for in health food shops, specialist shops and markets – and what to leave behind. Check out 'Ask Dr Agatston' on page 21 to find the answers to the questions asked most frequently about the South Beach Diet. Also included are real-life South Beach success stories and tips from people who have shared their motivating stories on the South Beach message boards at *www.prevention.com*. I hope they will inspire you to achieve your own success.

The diet has succeeded far beyond my expectations. It is responsible for millions of people losing weight safely and easily, and keeping it off while also improving their blood chemistries. My goal is to extend the benefits of the South Beach Diet still further. There are several ways to accomplish this. I have observed the best long-term results in those who have a good understanding of the few basic principles of the diet. This allows them to use flexibility and good judgement when making food choices in the various eating situations we all face: during travel, parties, stress, fatigue and when dining out. The other factor responsible for long-term compliance is the variety of foods and recipes available. This combats the repetition that leads to boredom on so many diets. Our goal for our heart patients as well as all of our readers is an overall healthier lifestyle leading to many permanent benefits.

In the meantime, I hope this cookbook helps you find the quality and variety of dishes to enable you to make the South Beach Diet the lifestyle it was intended to be.

WHAT IS THE SOUTH BEACH DIET?

Enjoying good food is a pleasure.

Eating is necessary for survival, of course, but it is also one of the great joys of life. We so love eating that we give our meals a social function. We enjoy our families and friendships around tables laden with good things to eat.

But our pleasure has also become our peril. Our relationship with food – or, rather, our excessive appetites for certain foods – is today, in many cases, hazardous to our health. If you've been following the news recently, you know what I'm talking about – skyrocketing obesity, which is associated with heart disease, cancer, strokes and diabetes, as a result of our unhealthy eating habits.

For years, we were taught by the experts that maintaining proper weight required sacrifice – that the only way to stay lean and mean was to give up many of the foods we loved. Millions of us started that challenging journey to good health but didn't necessarily get there. Many popular diets are geared to short-term weight loss and are clearly inappropriate for long-term weight control. In contrast, the South Beach Diet was developed to prevent heart attacks and strokes by improving our blood chemistries and trimming our waistlines. This means adopting a healthy lifestyle, not just looking for a quick fix.

Finding the *Real* Problem

Why has there been so much confusion about diet? It has largely been because, through new research, new information has been brought to light that has changed the conventional wisdom on how our bodies process food. The important effects of fibre, the glycaemic index (how fast a food raises our blood sugar) and the good fats, and the syndrome of pre-diabetes on weight and on health were simply not appreciated until recently.

But diets also failed because they didn't take into account how the average human being operates. The weight loss regimes were often impractical, cumbersome, unnatural and severe. They required us to abandon for ever the joys of eating a wide variety of good foods in amounts sufficient to satisfy our hunger and please our tastebuds.

I had a front-row view of how our misconceptions about nutrition and weight loss led us astray. As a cardiologist, my primary interest has been the prevention of heart disease. My proudest achievement thus far has been my role in the development of a heart scan protocol that uses rapid CT (computerized tomography technology) – which can, in minutes, easily and painlessly detect the build-up of arteriosclerosis in the walls of arteries years before it causes a heart attack or stroke. Around the world, the measure of coronary calcium (or plaque, as you might know it) is referred to as the Agatston Score.

That technology has saved many lives by detecting problems that would otherwise go unseen and finding them early enough to treat them without surgery. While this test can detect problems early, it cannot in itself prevent heart disease. But lifestyle changes, including proper diet and exercise, as well as certain medications, can prevent heart attacks. In this realm, I was stymied. Like other cardiologists, I urged my patients to lose weight and cut their cholesterol levels by going on the low-fat diet prescribed by the American Heart Association and other experts. But it didn't work as planned. Some patients went the low-fat route but didn't lose much weight at all. A few would diet religiously and exercise as they were instructed, lose the extra pounds, and feel fine. But then they'd grow tired of always feeling hungry, or they'd miss their favourite foods, or their will-power would just wear down. At that point, they'd start cheating here and there, and before we knew it, all the excess weight was back. In many cases, they'd end up heavier than before they started to diet. Too-rapid weight loss associated with crash diets actually lowers our metabolism and predisposes us to yo-yo dieting. In fact, the failures of low-fat, high-carb plans as well as rapid weight loss strategies have been well-documented in study after study.

Despite the lack of scientific proof that it worked, the low-fat regime became our weight loss gospel. We were lectured about the evils of meat, eggs, cheese, fats and oils. In response, food manufacturers began developing an entirely new category of products labelled 'low-fat' – which included everything from cakes and biscuits to salad dressings and crisps (potato chips). The foods *were* lower in fats, just as advertised. There was just one problem: the fats had been replaced by 'processed' carbohydrates – various forms of sugar for the most part, either white sugar itself or fructose, corn syrup, glucose syrup, honey, molasses, and modified starches bereft of fibre and nutrients.

In response, people felt free to eat these products with gusto. Unfortunately, I was one of those people consuming low-fat goodies – what a mistake! We had no idea that we were taking in more sugars and starches than ever before, and that this was causing rapid, large swings in our blood sugars that made us hungry again soon after we finished a meal or a snack. The international epidemic of obesity and diabetes was the result.

The 'Good Fats'

Because of my frustration with the low-fat, high-carb approach, and because I witnessed some successes with other high-saturated-fat, low-carb diets, I began my own study of the nutrition and weight loss literature. I wanted to find a healthy eating plan I could offer to my patients, something that would allow them to eat well but also to lose weight and improve their blood chemistries.

It soon became clear that the low-fat plan was fatally flawed. The bad fats – the so-called saturated ones, which exist mainly in animal products such as fatty meats, butter, cream and cheeses – *did* contribute to obesity, to some extent. But not nearly as much as we had been led to think. Their main health hazard was that they contributed to high levels of cholesterol and triglycerides in the blood, which in turn led to cardiovascular disease. As a cardiologist, that concerned me.

But there are also good fats, in particular olive oil, rapeseed (canola) oil, omega-3 fish oils, and the oils found in most nuts. These fats are not bad. They are not neutral. They are actually good for us. They help prevent heart attacks and strokes and also help our sugar and insulin metabolism, leading to better long-term weight control.

The 'Good Carbs'

As I studied, I learned that just as you cannot lump all fats together, neither can you condemn all carbohydrates. Just as there are good fats and bad fats, there are also good carbs and bad carbs. More precisely, there is a whole spectrum of carbohydrates, from very bad, to not so bad, to pretty good and, finally, very good. A well-rounded diet makes good use of good carbs.

There has never been any question about the benefits of eating carbs such as vegetables, beans and fruit. But back when the anti-fat gospel still held sway, we were instructed that even the starchiest refined carbohydrates – white bread, white pasta, potatoes and white rice – were healthy. In fact, however, these foods undermined our best efforts to lose weight.

All carbohydrates, even the healthiest vegetables, contain sugars. Starches, such as those found in potatoes, rice and wheat flour, are merely chains of sugar molecules. In the course of digestion, our bodies extract those sugars and put them to good use, providing us with necessary energy. Without sugars, we would die.

But before we can access those sugars, our digestive systems must separate them from the fibre that good carbs – such as vegetables and whole grains – also contain. That fibre slows down the digestive process, which is a good thing. It means that the sugars are released gradually into our bloodstreams. When that happens, the pancreas gets the signal and begins producing insulin. It is insulin's job to transport that blood sugar into our cells, where it can be burned for immediate energy or stored for later use.

Something very different takes place when we eat carbs that contain little or none of their original fibre, however. When that happens, our digestive systems begin processing all the sugars rapidly. As a result, the level of blood sugar – glucose – rises sharply, prompting the pancreas to release a large amount of insulin at once. In fact, the pancreas may actually over-react and send forth more insulin than is needed. That, in turn, causes a sharp drop in the level of glucose in the blood.

You are unaware of all this happening inside your body, but the fact is that you do sense it in an indirect way. That dramatic rise and fall of blood sugar creates cravings for more food. Your hunger is merely a response to changes in blood chemistry brought about by your metabolism. This par-ticular sensation drives you to want more food sooner than you would otherwise. And the craving is for more carbs.

The propensity of a food to cause swings in blood sugar is known as the glycaemic index (GI). It was developed in the 1980s by Dr David Jenkins, of the University of Toronto. This important concept was not available to the developers of earlier diets. The GI is a system that ranks foods by how quickly they cause blood sugar to rise when tested against 50 grams of glu-cose, which has a GI of 100. If the GI of food X is 50 per cent, then it raises blood sugar only 50 per cent as fast as glucose does. While we always assumed that table sugar raises your blood sugar faster than a white potato, Dr Jenkins's glycaemic index taught us that it doesn't. Why is this so impor-tant? The faster your blood sugar goes up after a meal, the faster it falls. In fact, after high-glycaemic-index meals, your blood sugar is likely to peak rapidly and then dive to a level lower than where it started. This blood sugar roller-coaster results in a range of feelings including irresistible cravings, severe fatigue, sleepiness, headaches and anxiety.

Once this phenomenon – known as reactive hypoglycaemia – occurs, you will typically grab the first carbohydrates available that will raise your blood sugar. Because the foods that raise your blood sugar the fastest are the ones that relieve your symptoms the fastest, they are what you reach for. This kicks off a vicious cycle. It takes some time for your body to recog-nize that its blood sugar level has normalized, but during this period you continue eating because you don't yet feel satisfied. So, without realizing it, you overeat, which leads to further swings in blood sugar, and the cycle repeats. This pattern is responsible for the developed world's epidemic of obesity and diabetes.

These facts of human metabolism have always been true. But the way our bodies process food is at odds with today's emphasis on quick, convenient and easy cooking. Virtually all of the fibre has been removed from everything made from white flour, for instance. That means most commercially made breads, biscuits and pies – anything that is baked. Many desserts and cakes fall into this category too. The same is true for breakfast cereals, even some of those that claim to be healthy, such as instant and quick-cooking porridge. Even rice has been processed for easy cooking – the removal of the fibre is why it can be ready so quickly.

In the case of grains, most of the fibre is found in the outer part of the grain, which also contains important vitamins and minerals; when you remove fibre, you remove those nutrients as well. This is why these carbs have been called 'empty calories'. Other than calories, they give us nothing else that our bodies require for optimal functioning. The fibre is also the element that slows the digestion of the carbohydrates. It encourages a slow, steady supply of sugar (energy) to our bodies, allowing us to function well for long periods without symptoms of hypoglycaemia.

Reversing the Trend

How do we set about reversing the obesity epidemic? As I mentioned, bad carbs are everywhere. They go into the most convenient foods, all the snacks that have become such a ubiquitous part of contemporary eating. Some people have a weakness for salty snacks, such as crisps or pretzels, which contain lots of bad carbs. Others have a sweet tooth, driving them to eat chocolate, ice cream, cakes or biscuits. Some people are beset by cravings for bread, pasta, potatoes, or rice. Whatever the craving, the result is the same: we overwhelm our systems with frequent infusions of highly processed carbohydrates and our bodies respond with urges for more. It's a strange phenomenon in that the food we eat, rather than satisfying our hunger, actually creates more hunger of its own.

Once this physiology became clear, an anti-carbohydrate camp rose up among some diet experts. Suddenly, all carbs were being blamed as the primary cause of obesity. In truth, a diet that's too low in carbohydrates will be lacking in nutrients, natural vitamins and dietary fibre – all of which are necessary for optimal health.

What's more, people enjoy eating carbohydrates. To give up foods such as bread, pasta, rice, and even fruit and some vegetables, seemed to be a terrible mistake. And by this point, we had all suffered enough under weight loss plans that required us to give up foods we loved. It is possible to eat carbs, even bread and rice and so on, as long as the grains have not been overly processed. If the whole grain is still present, carbs can be eaten by people watching their weight.

If you eat the right fats, like the kinds found in olive oil, nuts, avocados and omega-3 fish oils, you can lose weight and improve your health. And good fats make our food taste good.

The South Beach Diet: Striking the Balance

This was when it dawned on me that a healthy diet would be neither low-fat nor low-carb. Those extremes had caused, rather than cured, our obesity problem. A sound weight loss plan would make the distinction between good and bad fats and carbs. It would allow dieters to eat enough of the good carbs and fats, with plenty of natural vitamins and nutrients, so that no one would really miss the bad.

That was the first principle of the South Beach Diet.

The diet would make ample use of the foods that taste good and satisfy hunger: meat, poultry, seafood and vegetables, all cooked using good fats such as extra virgin olive oil and made flavourful with herbs, spices and the right sauces.

Another principle was that the food would have to be served in portions large enough to satisfy normal hunger. No one can go through life constantly feeling hunger pangs. That's why the South Beach Diet recommends that you eat three meals a day (breakfast, lunch and dinner), with a snack mid-morning and mid-afternoon.

As a chocoholic, I understand the importance of dessert. Because the South Beach Diet is meant to allow you to eat as naturally as possible, it includes desserts, even in the strictest phase. I think we've included some excellent dessert recipes in this book – dishes that taste great but can be enjoyed without falling off the weight-loss wagon. Many of the dessert recipes are fruit-based and replace sugar with a no-calorie sugar substitute. When possible, the fats are healthy ones rather than the saturated fats or trans fats that can lead to health problems.

The South Beach Diet programme is structured into three phases. The first, most restrictive, phase lasts for two weeks. It eliminates all starches including breads, rice, pasta and baked goods. It also restricts sugars, including all fruits and – sorry folks – no alcohol. The next chapter gives more details about the many things you can eat, as well as those you can't. You move on to the second phase to reach your target weight. In Phase 2 you add back starches in the form of whole grains, sugars in the form of low-glycaemic fruits, and alcohol with meals. Once you've reached your goal weight, you begin the third phase. At this point, the diet has become a lifestyle – a new way of eating that permits you to have the foods you like and still maintain your health and keep the weight off. You remain aware of what you learned in the first two phases, choosing a sweet potato instead of a white potato, brown rice instead of white, and wholegrain bread instead of white bread. In other words, you have learned the pecking order of the various classes of carbohydrates and how to apply it to your everyday life.

An important key to turning the South Beach Diet from a diet pro-gramme into a lifestyle is to have a great variety of foods and recipes that are simple and delicious. This cookbook will provide you with more than 200 choices to keep your meals fresh and exciting.

Here's to your health and bon appétit!

STOCKING THE SOUTH BEACH DIET KITCHEN

Changing how you eat will require some changes in how you shop, too. In fact, it will transform your kitchen, because that is the arena where dieters either succeed or fail. (I was going to say it's where you win or lose, except that in this particular contest, when you lose, you win!) Anyway, your store cupboards, refrigerator and freezer should look quite a bit different – vastly improved, of course – once you're on the South Beach Diet.

I can't emphasize enough the importance of having the right foods around the house, and not having the wrong ones. When I talk to people who have wavered on the diet, I hear the same basic story over and over again: 'I got home from work late, I was starving, and there were no vegetables in the refrigerator – so I microwaved some frozen chips instead.' Or, 'There was no sugar-free jelly, so I had a biscuit.' Or, 'I ran out of almonds so I ate some trail mix, washed down with a soft drink.' The South Beach Diet allows you a wide variety of delicious foods. You won't have to count calories or measure the quantities you consume. But it is important to steer clear of the truly unhealthy items that will undermine your success.

Even when you try, it's not always going to be the easiest thing to do.

For example, when one member of a couple goes on the diet and the other does not, a simple thing like a loaf of bread can become a battleground – the dieter wishes it would disappear, while the partner needs it for his or her daily sandwich. In one household I know, the wife has banished all bread, and the husband now goes out every afternoon to buy a single fresh roll for lunch. Dieters with children have an especially challenging time – no parent wants to deprive the kids of their little treats, but you may find it impossible to resist raiding the biscuit tin yourself. Will-power is needed, of course, though if you can get the children to love no-added-sugar lollies, you'll all be better off.

Maintaining a South Beach Diet-friendly kitchen is imperative if you're going to adopt healthy eating habits and lose excess weight. This chapter is a guide to what groceries you'll need to buy before you begin the diet. The list contains foods that are acceptable in Phase 1 – the initial, strict phase – and also in Phases 2 and 3, the less restrictive stages. I want to help you to create a healthy, balanced, well-appointed kitchen – a place where you can eat well *and* lose weight in the coming weeks or months.

You don't need to go out and buy every single item listed here; let your personal tastes be your guide. Your goal should be simply to stock up on the foods you like to eat. If you fill up on good foods, you won't have the need (or even the room) for anything else. Everything here should be available in any well-stocked supermarket. If you can't find a particular item where you shop, you can skip it and replace it with something else.

Cleaning Out the Kitchen Cupboards

Before you start that shopping trip, however, you may need to clear some space in your kitchen. So first, go through your cupboards, refrigerator and freezer and rid them of the foods that do not fit in the South Beach Diet. Some items can be packed away during the first two weeks on the diet, after which they will be allowed once more. Other goodies – the really troublesome ones – should probably just vanish forever. After the first phase of the diet, I promise, you will not miss them.

The list that follows contains many of the foods that you'll need to eliminate during Phase 1 of the South Beach Diet as well as some foods that are off-limits for Phase 2 as well. The list is very comprehensive, but it's impossible to list every food that dieters should avoid. Here's one good rule of thumb: if, among the first three ingredients, you see sugar in any form – meaning sugar (sucrose) itself and also fructose, maltose, dextrose, or anything with the suffix -*ose* – that food is almost certainly off-limits. During Phase 1, anything made with flour is taboo. After that, anything made with white flour is off-limits. Wholewheat (wholemeal) flour is better for you, but even then, you should not be eating baked goods with less than 2 grams of dietary fibre per serving.

So before you start Phase 1 of the diet, go through your kitchen and remove the following items:

Baked goods: this means all breads, cakes, biscuits, crackers, muffins, pastries and waffles. Even the healthiest breads made with wholemeal flour must go during Phase 1.

Cereals: all varieties of cereals are off-limits during the first two weeks of the diet. That includes the healthy ones that are high in fibre and with no added sugar, like porridge, bran flakes and kashi. The carbs in many commercial cereals cause a steep rise in blood sugar, which creates cravings for more carbs. Healthy high-fibre cereals reappear in Phase 2.

Dairy products: whole (full-fat) milk is banned in all phases of the South Beach Diet because of the saturated fats it contains. Cheeses and butter are severely limited.

Drinks: all fruit juices are banned for the first two weeks of the plan. All soft drinks containing sugar, fructose or glucose syrup are also forbidden.

Also for Phase 1, all alcoholic beverages are off-limits. That includes beer, cocktails, whisky, wine and wine coolers.

Fats and oils: as you clean out your kitchen, get rid of any solid vegetable fats, lard, duck or goose fat and beef dripping.

Fish and shellfish: there's no need to get rid of any fish. All fish are OK, canned or fresh. The oily ones – anchovies, mackerel, salmon and sardines – are especially recommended for the healthy omega-3 oils they contain.

Flour: all flour is taboo for Phase 1. That includes bread and cake mixes, pancake and waffle mixes. Cornmeal (polenta) is also not permitted.

Fruit: all fruit is forbidden during Phase 1. You'll reintroduce fruits to your diet two weeks from now, but until then, they have to go. Not only do they contain a lot of sugar, but they stimulate hunger, too. Same for any fruit products – jellies, jams and dried fruits, including raisins. Of course, any frozen foods containing fruit or fruit juice are also forbidden during Phase 1.

Meat and poultry: the South Beach Diet makes plentiful use of meat and poultry, but certain types are off-limits. Anything processed using sugars – glazed, honey-roast or maple-cured ham and bacon, for instance – is forbidden on all phases. When buying processed products, be sure to check the ingredients list. If you find any form of sugar in there, put it back. Pâté and offal such as liver and kidneys are forbidden, too. Most sausages are off-limits in all phases due to the saturated fats they contain.

Get rid of all fatty cuts of meat, including spare ribs and shoulder of lamb.

During Phase 1, fatty poultry such as duck and goose shouldn't be on the menu. Dark-meat chicken and turkey (legs and wings) are higher in fat than white (breast) meat and also are not allowed. Processed poultry, such as chicken nuggets, is forbidden in all phases.

Pasta: any kind of pasta is gone for Phase 1, even wholewheat.

Rice: rice of all varieties, even brown, is off-limits for the first two weeks.

Sauces, dressings and seasonings: barbecue sauces, ketchup and any other condiment or sauce made with glucose syrup, molasses, honey or sugar is banned. Even low-fat or fat-free condiments, such as mayonnaise, salad dressings and the like are off-limits. Surprised? In these products, the fat is usually replaced by refined carbohydrates. Get rid of any commercially made salad dressing that contains sugars (including fructose) or carbs, fat-free dressings included. Dressings made with olive oil and vinegar are fine; no-carb, sugar-free dressings are OK as well.

Most commercial teriyaki sauce and many chilli sauces are forbidden because of their sugar content. Chutney, sweet pickles and relish are also banned.

Snacks: all packaged snacks are off-limits, both the salty variety (crisps/potato chips, cheese puffs, popcorn, pretzels, tortilla chips and so on) and the sweet kind (biscuits, pies and the rest).

If we could just cut all processed foods from our diet, our weight would drop, and our overall health would improve. Processed carbs are problematic because the fibre, minerals and vitamins have been removed.

The type of carbs in these salty or sweet snacks causes a steep rise in blood sugar, which creates cravings for more carbs. Processed carbs are sometimes labelled as 'fortified' or 'vitamin-enriched' because of the manufacturers' attempt to restore some of the lost nutrients. But you can't replace natural vitamins with artificial ones and get the same health benefits. Additionally, many commercially prepared snack foods contain trans fats (hydrogenated vegetable oils, in other words oils that have been processed to turn them into solid fats).

Soup: rid your kitchen of all powdered soups, because many contain trans fats. You can have canned or fresh bean soups and clear broth (consommé) in any phase as long as they are not made with cream or butter and don't include pasta, rice or potatoes.

Sweeteners: all sweeteners, except sugar substitutes, are off-limits in Phase 1. This includes white sugar, brown sugar, honey, molasses, golden and maple syrup.

Vegetables: believe it or not, even a few vegetables must go for Phase 1. Potatoes are the biggest no-no – even boiled. Your digestive system immediately breaks the starches down into sugars, which end up as stored excess weight. Potatoes also create cravings for more bad carbs. For Phase 1, this includes sweet potatoes and yams.

Sweetcorn is also forbidden for now, along with beetroot, butternut squash, pumpkin and other winter squashes. All are turned quickly into sugars and stimulate hunger pangs. Even carrots and green peas are out of bounds for the first two weeks. Go through your freezer and get rid of any frozen foods that contain these vegetables.

The South Beach Shopping List

These are the items you're encouraged to enjoy on the South Beach Diet. I've broken this list into two sections. The first details the foods to enjoy in Phase 1, the most restrictive two weeks of the diet. The second lists the foods to eat in Phase 2. You don't need a list for Phase 3. This is how you'll eat for the rest of your life, and you'll know enough about the plan to make the right choices.

Phase 1 Shopping

Baked goods: steer clear of all baked goods during the entire two weeks of Phase 1.

Cereals: no cereals are allowed in Phase 1.

Dairy: in Phase 1, avoid whole milk, whole-milk yogurt and full-fat ice cream. You can have skimmed milk, fat-free natural yogurt, virtually fat-free cottage cheese and fromage frais, but no more than two servings a day. You can also use low-fat natural soya milk as a dairy substitute.

As for cheese, you can have pretty much any reduced-fat variety. That doesn't mean you can eat as much cheese as you like, but one or two small servings a day are fine. A good rule of thumb is to stick with cheeses containing no more than 6 g of fat per serving (if the nutrition information says there are 24 g of fat in 100 g of cheese, you should be OK). Feta cheese is a good choice, because the regular kind is so full of flavour that you don't need to use much.

Drinks: regular, caffeinated coffee is allowed, but no more than two cups a day, because caffeine has been found to stimulate insulin production. Decaf is permitted without limits. Tea is allowed, with the same qualifications. Green tea is unrestricted: it makes a refreshing drink and contains healthy antioxidants.

Obviously, water is fine. Flavoured waters are all right, too, as long as they don't have calories. Check the labels to be sure there's no sugar added. Soda water and low-calorie (sugar-free) tonic water are OK.

Diet soft drinks and low-calorie iced teas are all fine. Tomato juice, V8 and similar vegetable juice cocktails are allowed.

Eggs: eggs are allowed in Phase 1, unless you have dangerously high cholesterol. In truth, eggs aren't nearly as bad as we once thought – they raise the level of the good cholesterol as much as the bad, and they are a terrific source of natural vitamin E. If your doctor has advised you against eating eggs, ask him or her about using an egg substitute.

Fish and shellfish: all fresh fish, including oily fish such as herring, salmon, trout, tuna and mackerel are allowed. Smoked salmon, canned salmon, canned tuna, fresh or canned sardines and smoked fish are all OK. Shellfish such as mussels, crab, lobster and prawns are all permitted on the diet. Like meat, fish must be prepared in a healthy way – not breaded and definitely not deep-fried. Fish can be steamed, roasted, grilled, sautéed or baked.

Flour: avoid all flour in Phase 1.

Fruit: avoid all fruit and fruit juices in Phase 1.

Meat and poultry: most meats are permitted. They're a main source of protein, and if you choose carefully, you won't be overdoing the saturated fats. Meat is also good because it satisfies hunger so well. It should always be prepared using healthy methods, though, such as grilling, baking, roasting, or sautéing – but never deep-frying. When sautéing, use moderate amounts of healthy fats, such as extra virgin olive oil or rapeseed (canola) oil.

Sirloin, fillet and topside are the leanest cuts of beef and are all permitted; rump and T-bone steaks are fine as long as you cut off all the fat, and you can also enjoy lean stewing steak and extra-lean mince. For pork, fillet tenderloin, leg joints and lean, well-trimmed loin chops are acceptable. Lean boiled ham is OK at this stage, too. Back bacon is fine, but streaky is out. Veal chops and cutlets are acceptable, as is leg or loin of lamb, well trimmed of fat. Venison and other game meats are fine.

When buying cold meats, basically anything fat-free or low-fat is good. Boiled ham is fine, but any ham cured or processed using honey or sugar is not. Pastrami can be acceptable, as long as you can find a lean variety. Sliced turkey and chicken breast are fine, too.

For poultry, chicken breast, turkey breast, guinea fowl, ostrich and game birds such as pheasant and partridge are all fine – but don't eat the skin.

For breakfast, lean back bacon and turkey bacon are fine. Sausages are generally high in saturated fats – and low-fat varieties are often made with refined carbs. But you can use minced turkey breast to make your own sausages for breakfast – see page 54.

If you use meat substitutes, tofu, tempeh and any other soya-based product is allowed in all phases of the diet. Veggie burgers are also allowed.

Oils and fats: extra virgin olive oil, rapeseed (canola) oil, flaxseed oil, peanut (groundnut) oil, sesame oil and walnut oil are all fine on all three phases, both for cooking and for salad dressings. (Most 'pure vegetable oil' sold in the UK and Australia is rapeseed (canola) oil – a quick look at the ingredients list will confirm this.) You will use far less oil in cooking if you spray it rather than pour it, and many of the recipes in this book call for cooking spray. There are various types of cooking spray available in the shops; choose olive oil rather than sunflower oil.

Sometimes only a buttery taste will do. Luckily, there are an increasing number of spreads with a buttery flavour that do not contain either saturated fats or trans fats (hydrogenated vegetable oils) – you will need to check the nutrition information panel carefully before you buy. Some low-fat spreads are made from hydrogenated vegetable oils, and if the fat content is less than 50% they cannot be used for cooking. Best of all are the spreads that actually lower cholesterol, such as Benecol and Proactiv (Take Control).

Pasta: no pasta is allowed in Phase 1.

Rice: no rice is allowed in Phase 1.

Sauces, dressings and seasonings: just about any herb, spice or seasoning is fine on this diet. In fact, I encourage you to use anything you like that enhances the flavour of food. If your healthy dishes taste great, you'll be less tempted to indulge in the unhealthy ones. Why not experiment with the myriad spices and seasonings available in your supermarket?

Try herbs like basil, oregano, thyme and parsley, or add a little heat with cumin, curry powder or chilli. Garlic is something you'll get lots of use from – you can buy it fresh, powdered, or puréed. Nutmeg, cinnamon and cloves will add aromatic warmth to a dish, while dill, mint and rosemary will add a striking freshness. Used alone or in combination, herbs and spices will breathe new life into any dish you make. Extracts, such as almond and vanilla, are great to add to your foods as well.

Any mustard (except honey mustard), mayonnaise, Tabasco and other hot-pepper sauces, horseradish, salsa, light soy sauce (preferably low-sodium) and Worcestershire sauce are legal in all phases, even 1 – but check the label before you buy, to be sure there's no sugar, glucose syrup or starch in the ingredients listed. See the recipes beginning on page 162 for some homemade condiments you'll love.

To dress your salads, choose any of the approved oils (rapeseed/canola, flaxseed, extra virgin olive oil, groundnut/peanut, sesame, or walnut) mixed with vinegar (such as balsamic or wine). Among the prepared dressings, Newman's Own Light Balsamic Vinaigrette and Newman's Own Olive Oil and Vinegar dressing are allowed, as is Cardini's Original Caesar Salad Dressing. In fact, just about any no-carb, sugar-free dressing will do.

Snacks: limit sweet treats to 75 calories (315 kilojoules) per day in Phase 1. Reach for sugar-free boiled sweets, no-added-sugar lollies, sugar-free jelly and sugar-free chewing gum. If you have a sweet tooth you can mix unsweetened cocoa powder with ricotta and sugar substitute to make a luxurious snack. If you like savoury snacks, you're allowed a few cherry tomatoes, radishes, sticks of celery or pepper (capsicum), with a tablespoon of nut butter, hummus or some low-fat cheese. A handful of olives is fine, too.

All types of nuts are fine in Phase 1 – even macadamias, which we used to think were unhealthy. Almonds are best for the nutrients they contain, but you should really limit consumption of nuts to about 30 g (1 oz) a day. Pumpkin and sunflower seeds are also good, healthy snacks.

Soups: clear soups and low-fat tinned bean soups are fine in Phase 1.

Sweeteners: you can use any no-calorie sugar substitute you like. Splenda (sucralose) has less of a bitter aftertaste than aspartame sweetener.

Vegetables: most vegetables are allowed on all phases of the diet. All the green ones can stay. Spinach and other leafy dark green vegetables are fine. The same is true for globe artichokes, asparagus, aubergines (eggplant), avocados, bean sprouts, beans (fresh, dried or tinned), broccoli, brussels sprouts, cabbage, cauliflower, celery, chickpeas, courgettes (zucchini), cucumber, fennel, leeks, lentils and split peas, lettuce, mangetouts (snow peas), mushrooms, onions, peppers (capsicums), radishes, spring onions, shallots, spaghetti squash, turnips, water chestnuts. Tomatoes are OK in Phase 1.

Phase 2 Shopping

After the first two weeks on the South Beach Diet, you'll enter the Phase 2 eating regime. In this second phase, you can enjoy all of the foods from Phase 1, plus some additions.

I always advise dieters to reintroduce carbohydrates gradually – maybe one piece of fruit a day, or a portion of brown rice or wholewheat pasta once or twice a week. If it's bread you want, you should be eating wholegrain varieties.

If you add more carbs back to your diet and notice that your weight loss stalls, you've probably gone too far. On the other hand, if you can eat a piece of bread every day without undermining your hard work, feel free.

In Phase 2, you can go out and buy these items:

Baked goods: this may be the most confusing aisle in the supermarket. You'll see various types of mixed grain and multigrain bread, which might lead you to think you're getting something healthy. But check the ingredients: if the first item on the list is not wholewheat (wholemeal) or another wholegrain, it's a no-no. Wholegrain bread is always available in health food shops. In general, look for bread with 100 per cent wholewheat flour as the first ingredient. Or try multigrain, oat and bran, rye and pumpernickel breads. Bread should contain at least 2.5 grams of dietary fibre per slice. (Pay extra attention here, because some manufacturers will give the information per serving, which may mean for two slices.)

There are quite a few flatbreads and crackers made with wholegrain wheat that are fine in Phases 2 and 3. Pitta bread is also acceptable after the first two weeks. Look for stoneground or wholewheat types. Small, wholegrain bagels are fine in Phase 2.

Overall, I suggest no more than one or two starches a day. It can be a slice of wholegrain bread with lunch and then a serving of brown rice with dinner. Maybe wholewheat pasta at one meal and a baked small sweet potato with another. Try to accompany all such carbs with a healthy protein, such as meat, fish or cheese. Fats will slow down the speed with which your body processes carbs, which is a good thing to do.

When buying breads and baked goods, beware of any hydrogenated and partially hydrogenated oils – they're all bad for your cardiovascular system.

Continue to avoid refined wheat (white) breads, rolls and bagels.

Cereals: stay away from instant or microwave oat cereals, but feel free to enjoy the old-fashioned kind you cook on the hob (stove). Some cold cereals are fine – Kellogg's All-Bran is a good one – but most of them contain too much sugar and too little fibre to be any good for you. Even muesli, despite its healthy reputation, usually has too much sugar. You'll see cereal labelled 'fat-free', but the fat never was the problem in cereal – it's the bad carbs and sugar.

Avoid cornflakes, even in Phase 2.

Dairy: the same rules as in Phase 1 apply.

Drinks: it's OK to have a daily glass or two of red or white wine and it's best to have wine with a meal because your blood sugar will rise less rapidly. But steer clear of any kind of beer: it raises blood sugar much faster than table sugar. Whisky, too, rapidly converts to sugar, and should also be avoided, as should cocktails. Continue to avoid all fruit juices and soft drinks made with sugar in Phase 2.

Fish and shellfish: it's still a good idea to enjoy lots of fish and shellfish, prepared in healthy ways.

Flour: in Phase 2, you can reintroduce wholewheat (wholemeal) flour. Whole wheat flour, buckwheat flour, rye flour and barley flour are just a few of the many varieties available in supermarkets. There are also flours made from soya beans and chickpeas (gram flour), which are extremely healthy.

Fruit: now it's OK to enjoy fresh fruit. Choose apples, apricots, blueberries, cherries, grapefruit, grapes, kiwi fruit, mangoes, orange- and green-skinned melons, oranges, peaches, pears, plums, raspberries and strawberries. You can also enjoy dried apricots, apple rings and prunes, but steer clear of other dried fruit as it raises blood sugar rapidly.

Even in Phase 2, avoid bananas, pineapple, raisins and sultanas, watermelon, canned fruit packed in juice or syrup, and all sugared jams.

Meat and poultry: the same meats and poultry you ate in Phase 1 are still great choices in Phase 2. Continue to avoid pâté and fatty poultry such as duck and goose.

Oils: continue using the same oils in Phase 2 that we used in Phase 1 in limited quantities.

Pasta: if it's made with wholewheat flour, it's approved after Phase 1.

Rice: white rice is forbidden during any phase; you'll be safer eating either basmati rice, brown rice, or wild rice (which isn't a rice at all – it's a seed). Steer clear of instant rice.

Breaking the Rules

You may be surprised to find that a handful of recipes in this book call for small quantities of ingredients that are either 'off limits' in a particular phase or 'off limits' on the diet in general. Some examples of this are a tablespoon of dry sherry in a Phase 1 beef and pepper salad, white flour as well as wholemeal flour in a Phase 3 quick bread, or white sugar in some of the Phase 3 desserts. When we include these foods, it's because they greatly enhance either the flavour or the texture of a dish, and since the total quantity – which is small to begin with – is spread out over several servings, you don't consume the full amount in your portion.

But just as importantly, these few recipes remind us that a little flexibility goes a long way in adapting the South Beach Diet as a lifestyle. If you stick to the nutritional guidelines of whichever phase you're on, an occasional small detour shouldn't have any lasting effect on your weight loss or overall health goals.

Sauces, dressings and seasonings: the sauce rules as in Phase 1 apply.

Snacks: in Phase 2, you may add chocolate back to your diet sparingly, choosing dark plain chocolate with a high percentage of cocoa solids. Enjoy sugar-free, fat-free desserts, too. Air-popped popcorn without oil is a great snack to add in Phase 2. Keep away from the biscuits and cakes, crisps (potato chips), pretzels and other salty and sweet snacks.

Soup: in Phase 2, you can have canned bean and vegetable soups, so long as there's no pasta, potatoes or other starches included. Powdered soups are always a bad idea – they contain too many carbs and may contain trans fats.

Sweeteners: after Phase 1, honey and molasses can come back in moderation, but other sugars should be for special occasions only.

Vegetables: at this point, you may reintroduce sweet potatoes, carrots, green peas and yams to your diet. Continue avoiding beetroot, sweetcorn and white potatoes. Again, start slowly and monitor what eating these vegetables does to your diet and your cravings.

Note: All spoon measures are level. 1 teaspoon = 5 ml; 1 tablespoon = 15 ml. For accuracy, invest in a set of measuring spoons.

ASK DR AGATSTON

As you might imagine, we get lots of questions about foods and methods of preparation. Here are some of the most commonly asked ones.

Is it all right to eat reheated leftovers from dinner for breakfast? I'm not a big fan of eggs.

Leftovers are fine for any meal, as long as they are consistent with the rules for your phase of the diet. It's probably not a great idea to start the day with fruit, pasta or rice, however. That's because these foods can stimulate cravings for more carbs later. But fish, meat or vegetables are great choices for breakfast.

Is every kind of bean allowed in all phases of the diet?

Most beans are allowed in all phases: they're good sources of nutrients and protein and they're delicious. Avoid canned beans that contain sugar or fat.

Aren't some shellfish – like lobster, for instance – bad for people on a diet or for those of us who have high cholesterol?

No! The amount of cholesterol in shellfish has always been exaggerated because the sterols they contain were misunderstood – they are chemically similar to cholesterol, but they actually help decrease cholesterol levels. Lobster has the same amount of cholesterol as skinless chicken breast. All shellfish are low in saturated fat and are not restricted on the diet.

What should I be using instead of butter for cooking and on top of bread or steamed vegetables?

In cooking, we suggest extra virgin olive oil if you want a rich flavour, or rapeseed (canola) oil for a lighter touch. Extra virgin olive oil is also delicious on bread. You can add garlic, a little grated cheese, or roasted peppers (capsicums) to the oil for flavour. Atop vegetables, try extra virgin olive oil and lemon instead of butter. There are also some good cholesterol-lowering vegetable-spread products to use in place of butter, on bread or anywhere else. Popular brands include Benecol and Proactiv (known as Take Control in the US). Avoid vegetable spreads that contain trans fats – the list of ingredients will include the words 'hydrogenated vegetable oil'.

I've tried modified carb diets before but always suffered with constipation as a result. Is there any way to avoid this on the diet?

Yes, there is. You need to maximize your fibre intake by eating plenty of whole grains and whole fruits and vegetables. In all phases, you can also take fibre supplements or psyllium to prevent constipation. Fibre supplements taken with meals actually help control blood sugar and insulin levels and can also help lower your cholesterol. Remember to drink at least 2 litres (3½ pints) of water every day.

Is it safe for children to follow the South Beach Diet?

The epidemic of obesity and diabetes has now extended to teenagers and even younger children. The South Beach Diet is the answer to this epidemic, and its principles are exactly the ones that should be applied to our children. The good fats, particularly omega-3 oils, are crucial for the development of young nervous systems, while trans fats (hydrogenated fats, which are found in many processed foods) are dangerous. The good carbs, including whole grains and whole fruits and vegetables, provide the vitamins, minerals and nutrients kids especially need. I believe that most children should begin with the Phase 2 eating plan, and you should always consult your child's doctor before putting your child on any diet plan.

Are tomatoes allowed?

Yes, they're fine in all phases, even though technically they are fruits. We even suggest tomato juice or V8 vegetable juice cocktail with breakfast.

Tomato and tomato sauces contain lycopene, which may help prevent prostate cancer.

Which sweeteners are all right for use in cooking and baking?

No-calorie sugar substitutes such as Splenda are fine in any phase. After Phase 1, try using apple sauce or apple purée, as long as it has no added sugar. Fruit juices are allowed in cooking, too, but in moderation. You can use a little honey or molasses to impart some of their flavour and moisture, beginning in Phase 2, but you should combine it with a sugar substitute.

Is there any difference between frozen vegetables and fresh?

There's no difference in terms of the diet. In fact, some frozen vegetables have more nutrients than fresh ones because they are blanched and frozen as soon as they're picked, whereas 'fresh' produce may sit around in transport or on shop shelves for several days before you eat it.

How do I know (other than by weighing myself) if I'm overdoing good carbs once I reintroduce them to my diet? Are there any other signs or symptoms?

The basic guide to success on the South Beach Diet is the disappearance of cravings. This should occur fairly early in Phase 1. If strong cravings for bread, potatoes and so on recur in Phase 2, you've probably been eating too many carbs, and you need to cut back. Weight loss during Phase 2 should be ½ to 1 kg (1 to 2 lb) a week. If loss has stalled, this is probably the result of too many bad carbs.

Is lamb all right on the diet?

Lamb does contain more saturated fat than beef or chicken, but it's allowed as long as it has been well-trimmed of fat. Leg and loin of lamb are the leanest cuts; chops should be a special treat.

I'm a sandwich addict. I also like the convenience of sandwiches. But I don't want to overdo bread by having two slices every day for lunch. Is there an alternative?

It's possible to make sandwiches without bread – take your ingredients, such as turkey, ham, or whatever, add mustard or mayonnaise, tomato and seasonings, and wrap it all up in a few lettuce leaves. You can compromise by using just one slice of wholegrain bread or a small wholewheat pitta.

Are nut butters allowed?

Yes, all are permitted and even encouraged because they're healthy and they taste good. But buy the kind with no added ingredients – health food shops and many supermarkets now sell almond, cashew and peanut butter that consist of the pure nuts with no additional sugars or fats.

Which pickles and relishes are allowed?

The sour varieties are fine, but not the sweet. Sugar is added to the vinegar used to make gherkins, and is often used in chutneys and pickles.

Can I have sushi on the diet?

Because of the sticky rice, sushi is for Phase 3 dieters only. But those in Phases 1 and 2 can feel free to eat sashimi, the raw fish without the rice.

What's the difference between whole milk, semi-skimmed (low-fat), skimmed and soya, in terms of the diet?

The sugar in dairy products takes the form of lactose, which is not harmful to your diet like normal table sugar. But whole milk also contains saturated fat, which is bad for your heart. Because milk is a good source of calcium, you're better off using low-fat dairy products. Soya milk is a good source of protein and is perfect for people who are lactose-intolerant or just don't like cow's milk. But check the label – some brands add more sugar (sometimes in the form of fruit juice) than others.

Is it OK to have sorbet or frozen yogurt for dessert?

Neither is a good choice as both contain a lot of sugar. Try sugar-free ice lollies or ice pops (ice blocks) instead. If you're going to break the diet, why not have a small scoop of real ice cream? That way, you won't be under the illusion that you've been virtuous. Try mixing it with healthy items such as fruit, or stir in some almonds, peanuts or walnuts.

Can I make my own sorbet using crushed ice, lemon juice and sugar substitute?

Sounds perfectly fine – you can't go wrong with those ingredients. But you should probably prepare it and eat it immediately, because with a little time in the freezer, it may turn into a solid rock of lemon ice.

When can I start eating chocolate again?

Even in Phase 1, you can make a dessert using unsweetened cocoa, ricotta cheese or virtually fat-free fromage frais, vanilla extract and sugar substitute. In Phase 2, you can have small amounts of dark chocolate, preferably in combination with other things, like strawberries. Try a tiny taste of it to finish off a meal – for example, two or three chocolate espresso beans, or a few squares of really good (high cocoa solids) dark chocolate. (The dark kind has less sugar than milk chocolate.) The key is to keep it under control.

Are olives all right? With pimientos?

They're perfectly fine – olives are as healthy as extra virgin olive oil, a good source of monounsaturated fat. The pimientos are simply red peppers (capsicums), and they are good, too.

Can I have commercial (unsweetened) breakfast cereal with semi-skimmed (low-fat) milk?

Not in Phase 1. In Phase 2 you can, but stick with cereals that are highest in fibre and lowest in sugar. Those made with whole grains are best. You should steer clear of cereals made from corn.

I love Mexican food, but I know the dishes are high in carbs. Is there a way to get around that?

Sure, if you can resist the tortilla chips that appear on the table, and then not order a burrito, enchilada, taco, tamale or tortilla. Rice is also not recommended for dieters on Phases 1 or 2. Try some of the salsa with vegetables instead of tortilla chips, and then stick to dishes without any kind of tortilla wrap. Mexican cuisine makes great use of meats and fish in flavourful sauces.

I love salty snacks, such as crisps (potato chips), tortilla chips, popcorn, pretzels, and the rest. Which of those is worst for dieters?

In terms of the bad carbs, pretzels are worst, followed by tortilla chips, potato crisps (which are also high in bad fats), and then packaged popcorn. We've got a terrific recipe for roasted chickpeas (see page 75) that can take the place of these items. Air-popped popcorn without butter can be eaten as a snack in Phase 2.

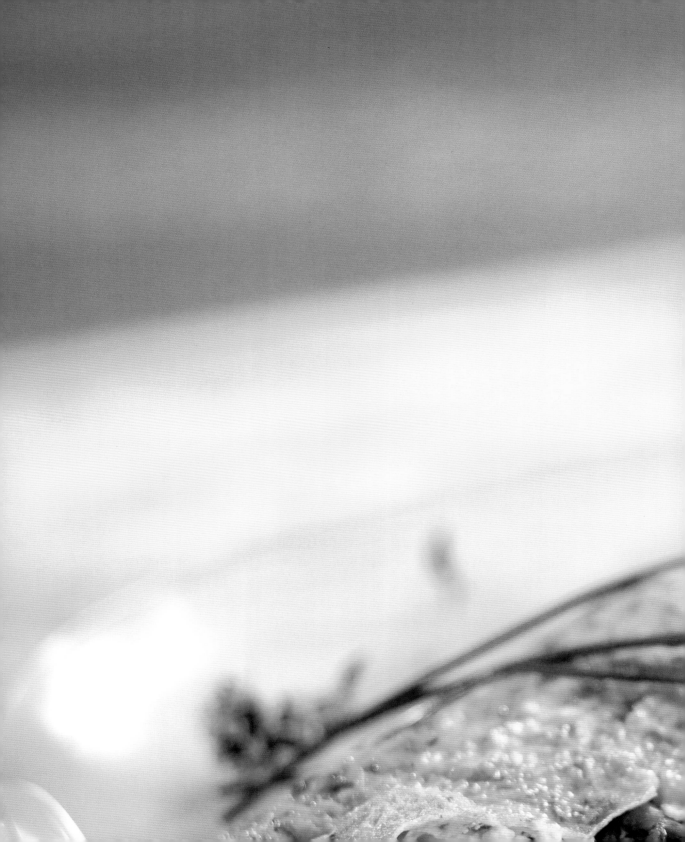

BREAKFASTS

In my medical practice, I've observed that a great many patients who say they never eat breakfast also suffer from obesity. Is there a connection? Quite possibly. Going too long without food can be a problem, because the resulting hunger pangs can cause you to overeat, usually the worst foods. That alone makes it important to start the day with a satisfying meal.

Bad breakfast habits may also set you up for trouble at lunchtime or later. One important study proved that starting the morning with processed carbohydrates — a bagel, say, or toast and marmalade — will stimulate cravings for more of the same throughout the day. The same research has shown that a breakfast based on good proteins and fats — like a cheese and vegetable omelette — will actually keep those urges away. Eggs, vegetables and lean meats are all healthy ways to start the day.

Oat Smoothie

If you're not a fan of strawberries, you can replace them with the berry of your choice in this quick and delicious breakfast shake.

375 g (13 oz)	strawberries, halved
230 g (8 oz)	fat-free natural yogurt
4	tablespoons dried skimmed milk
30 g (1 oz)	walnuts, chopped
3	tablespoons oat bran
1–2	tablespoons sugar substitute
90 g (3 oz)	crushed ice

In a blender or food processor, combine the strawberries, yogurt, dried milk, walnuts, oat bran, sugar substitute and ice. Blend until smooth and frothy.

Makes 4 servings

NUTRITION AT A GLANCE

Per serving: Energy 190 cals/795 kJ; 7 g fat (of which 1 g saturates), 10 g protein, 24 g carbohydrate (of which 16 g sugars), 2 g fibre, 121 mg sodium

Apricot Muffins

Rather than munching a sugar-packed bakery muffin, enjoy these healthy alternatives as an occasional breakfast in Phase 3. The soya in these muffins provides you with phytochemicals, protein and dietary fibre and has been proven to reduce 'bad' cholesterol.

250 g (9 oz)	wholemeal flour
30 g (1 oz)	soya flour
2	tablespoons sugar substitute
4	tablespoons sugar
1	tablespoon baking powder
1	teaspoon ground cinnamon
½	teaspoon ground nutmeg
	pinch of salt
1	egg, beaten
180 ml (6 fl oz)	soya milk
170 g (6 oz)	unsweetened apple sauce or purée
3	tablespoons rapeseed (canola) oil
10	ready-to-eat dried apricots, chopped

Preheat the oven to 200°C/400°F/gas 6. Coat a 12-cup non-stick muffin tin with cooking spray or line with paper cake cases.

In a large bowl, thoroughly combine the wholemeal and soya flours, sugar substitute, sugar, baking powder, cinnamon, nutmeg and salt. Make a hollow in the centre of the mixture and add the egg, soya milk, apple sauce, oil and apricots, stirring until moistened; do not overmix. Spoon the mixture into the prepared muffin tin.

Bake for 14 minutes, or until a skewer inserted into the centre of a muffin comes out clean. Leave to cool in the tin for about 10 minutes, then transfer to a rack to cool completely.

Makes 12 muffins

NUTRITION AT A GLANCE

Per muffin: Energy 155 cals/648 kJ; 4 g fat (of which 0.5 g saturates), 5 g protein, 26 g carbohydrate (of which 11 g sugars), 2.5 g fibre, 228 mg sodium

Wholesome Oat Muffins

Why not make a double batch of these healthy muffins and freeze half for later?

115 g (4 oz)	+ 2 tablespoons oats
240 ml (8 fl oz)	buttermilk
145 g (5 oz)	wholemeal flour
1½	teaspoons baking powder
½	teaspoon bicarbonate of soda
¼	teaspoon ground cinnamon
¼	teaspoon salt
75 g (2½ oz)	walnuts, chopped
80 ml (3 fl oz)	rapeseed (canola) oil
1	egg, beaten
2	tablespoons brown sugar
2	tablespoons sugar substitute, preferably brown
1	teaspoon vanilla extract

Preheat the oven to 220°C/425°F/gas 7. Coat a 12-cup non-stick muffin tin with cooking spray or line with paper cake cases.

In a small bowl, combine 115 g (4 oz) of the oats and the buttermilk. Leave to soak for 30 minutes.

In a medium bowl, combine the flour, baking powder, bicarbonate of soda, cinnamon, salt and walnuts.

In a large bowl, stir together the oil, egg, sugar, sugar substitute and vanilla extract until well blended. Stir in the oat mixture. Stir in the flour mixture until just combined; do not overmix. Spoon the batter into the prepared muffin tin, filling each cup about two-thirds full. Sprinkle the remaining 2 tablespoons oats over the muffins.

Bake for 11 to 15 minutes, or until a skewer inserted into the centre of a muffin comes out clean. Leave to cool in the tin for 5 minutes, then transfer to a rack to cool completely.

Makes 12 muffins

NUTRITION AT A GLANCE

Per muffin: Energy 159 cals/665 kJ; 6 g fat (of which 1 g saturates), 6 g protein, 22 g carbohydrate (of which 5 g sugars), 2 g fibre, 158 mg sodium

Apple Walnut Muffins

Chopped fresh apple flavours these moist muffins. If you really like cinnamon, you can add an extra ¼ to ½ teaspoon.

170 g (6 oz)	wholemeal flour
2	teaspoons baking powder
1	teaspoon bicarbonate of soda
1	teaspoon ground cinnamon
¼	teaspoon salt
180 ml (6 fl oz)	buttermilk
3	tablespoons rapeseed (canola) oil
2	tablespoons brown sugar
1–2	tablespoons sugar substitute
1	egg, beaten
1	medium apple, peeled and finely chopped
60 g (2 oz)	walnuts, chopped
1	teaspoon grated orange zest

Preheat the oven to 200°C/400°F/gas 6. Coat a 12-cup non-stick muffin tin with cooking spray or line with paper cake cases.

In a medium bowl, combine the flour, baking powder, bicarbonate of soda, cinnamon and salt.

In a large bowl, combine the buttermilk, oil, brown sugar, sugar substitute and egg. Stir in the flour mixture until just combined; do not overmix. Stir in the apple, walnuts and grated orange zest. Spoon the batter into the prepared muffin tin, filling each cup about two-thirds full.

Bake for 12 minutes, or until a skewer inserted into the centre of a muffin comes out clean. Leave to cool in the tin for 5 minutes, then transfer to a rack to cool completely.

Makes 12 muffins

NUTRITION AT A GLANCE
Per muffin: Energy 137 cals/573 kJ; 7 g fat (of which 0.5 g saturates), 4 g protein, 15 g carbohydrate (of which 6 g sugars), 1.5 g fibre, 195 mg sodium

Wholemeal Loaf

If you've had difficulty finding a bread that fits your new way of eating, you might want to try this simple wholemeal bread. It's easy to make and the results are delicious.

350 ml (12 fl oz)	warm water (use one part boiling water to two parts cold water)
2½	tablespoons extra virgin olive oil
400–455 g (14 oz–1 lb)	wholemeal bread flour
60 g (2 oz)	walnuts, chopped
1	teaspoon salt
1 sachet (7 g)	easy-bake yeast

In a large mixing bowl, using an electric mixer or a wooden spoon, combine the water, oil, wholemeal flour, walnuts, salt and yeast to form a rough dough. Let the dough stand for 15 to 20 minutes.

Place the dough on a lightly floured board and knead for 10 to 15 minutes, until the dough is smooth and elastic; add a little more flour if it feels sticky.

Coat a 1 kg (2 lb) loaf tin with cooking spray. Preheat the oven to 230°C/450°F/gas 8.

Place the dough in the tin, pressing it into the corners, and cover it with a clean damp cloth. Let the dough rise in a warm place for 30 minutes, or until it has doubled in size.

Place the tin in the centre of the oven. Bake for about 30 minutes. The loaf is ready when it sounds hollow if you knock on the bottom of it. Turn the bread out onto a rack and leave to cool.

Makes 16 slices

NUTRITION AT A GLANCE
Per slice: Energy 129 cals/540 kJ; 5 g fat (of which 0.5 g saturates), 4 g protein, 19 g carbohydrate (of which 0.5 g sugars), 2 g fibre, 147 mg sodium

A Guide to Grains and Baked Goods

The biggest adjustment for most people on the South Beach Diet is having to change their relationship with carbohydrates. Many carbs are good for you, and they are an important part of this regime. Vegetables contain carbs, and you'll eat them in abundance. You'll enjoy fruit, too, once you've gone beyond the first two weeks of the programme. But to many people, carbs often mean comfy, cosy treats like breads and baked goods.

Some of these carbs – the highly processed packaged ones – are going to have to become 'once in a great while' treats. There's virtually no way to eat them as often as you used to and still lose weight. Nearly all the fibre and nutrients have been removed in the manufacturing process, leaving only the sugars and starches. They cause you to store excess weight, and they create cravings for even more bad carbs.

But I recognize that a normal diet will probably include bread, and even muffins or pancakes once in a while. Luckily, you can go on eating these foods while on the South Beach plan. You may even be able to use some of your favourite recipes. They will simply require a little adaptation – replacing the bad grains, which have low fibre, with better ones.

Take bread, for example. The kind that you buy in supermarkets and in most bakeries is made with fortified flour, from which the outer part of the grain has been removed. Once that part has been stripped away, the fibre and many of the nutrients go with it. A single slice of white or brown bread has the equivalent impact on your blood sugar of a tablespoon of pure white sugar, straight from the bowl. Many people eat that bread with breakfast, lunch and dinner. You can imagine the effect of six or more slices a day on your attempts to lose weight.

If you take any recipe and replace at least some of the white flour with wholemeal flour – preferably stoneground – or rye or soya flour, you increase the amount of fibre and decrease the degree to which it raises your blood sugar level. You still won't be able to consume six slices a day, but bread will be back on your eating plan without wrecking your diet. The same is true for muffins and pancakes.

You can usually find several kinds of flour in a supermarket or health food shop, nearly all of which are better for you than the standard white kind. Here's how to get bread and baked goods back into your diet, once you've reached Phase 3.

Bread You can take any recipe for white bread and replace half the flour with wholemeal flour. It's that simple. Spelt flour, milled from an ancient variety of wheat, makes tasty bread; it rises quickly, so you will need to reduce the proving time if you are adapting a recipe based on regular wheat flour.

Rye flour makes bread with an interesting, slightly sour flavour. Because rye flour is denser than white flour, you should increase the amount of yeast so that the bread rises properly. If you use light rye flour, replace half the white flour with it. If using medium rye flour, replace one-third of the white flour. If using dark rye flour, replace no more than one-quarter of the white flour in your bread recipe. There's even something called dark rye meal, which will give you pumpernickel bread – dark, dense and very tasty.

You can also make bread using buckwheat flour or oat flour: replace one-quarter of the white flour with it, and increase the yeast slightly, too. If you can't find oat flour in your health food shop, simply process rolled oats (traditional porridge oats) in a blender or food processor until they form a fine meal.

Soya flour has a lot of good protein: replace up to one-eighth of the white flour with soya flour. You must also increase the amount of liquid in the recipe and reduce the oven temperature by 10–15°C/25°F. You may also need to add a little more yeast to make sure the loaves rise properly.

'Quick breads' and muffins 'Quick bread' means any kind made using baking powder and bicarbonate of soda instead of yeast. The dough doesn't rise – you just bake the batter. You can simply replace half the white flour with wholemeal. Wholemeal flour is coarser than white flour, so do not try to sift it. Quick breads made with wholemeal flour will have a nutty flavour and may have slightly less volume than those made with white flour.

You can make muffins with oat bran instead of flour, too. You can also use barley flour, which has a mild taste, or oat flour, which is especially good in biscuits.

Pancakes Buckwheat is used to make the *galettes de sarrasin* of Brittany and the Russian *blini*. If you're making pancakes from scratch, replace up to one-fifth of the white flour in your favourite pancake recipe with buckwheat flour.

You can also make pancakes using wholemeal flour or oat bran.

Breakfast Popovers with Parmesan

These popovers, like miniature Yorkshire puddings, are great for breakfast with family or friends. For variety, you can swap the Parmesan for other hard cheeses, such as Pecorino or aged Manchego.

2	eggs
145 g (5 oz)	wholemeal flour
270 ml (9 fl oz)	skimmed milk
1	tablespoon trans-fat-free butter substitute, melted
4	tablespoons freshly grated Parmesan cheese

Preheat the oven to 200°C/400°F/gas 6. Coat 8 individual Yorkshire pudding tins or custard cups with cooking spray.

Whisk the eggs in a medium bowl. Add the flour, milk and butter substitute and whisk until the ingredients are combined. Stir in 3 tablespoons of the cheese.

Divide the batter among the prepared tins and sprinkle with the remaining cheese. Place the tins on a large baking sheet.

Bake for 30 minutes, or until the popovers are puffed and golden. Remove from the tins and serve hot.

Makes 8 popovers

NUTRITION AT A GLANCE
Per popover: Energy 142 cals/594 kJ; 6.5 g fat (of which 3 g saturates), 8 g protein, 14 g carbohydrate (of which 2 g sugars), 1 g fibre, 137 mg sodium

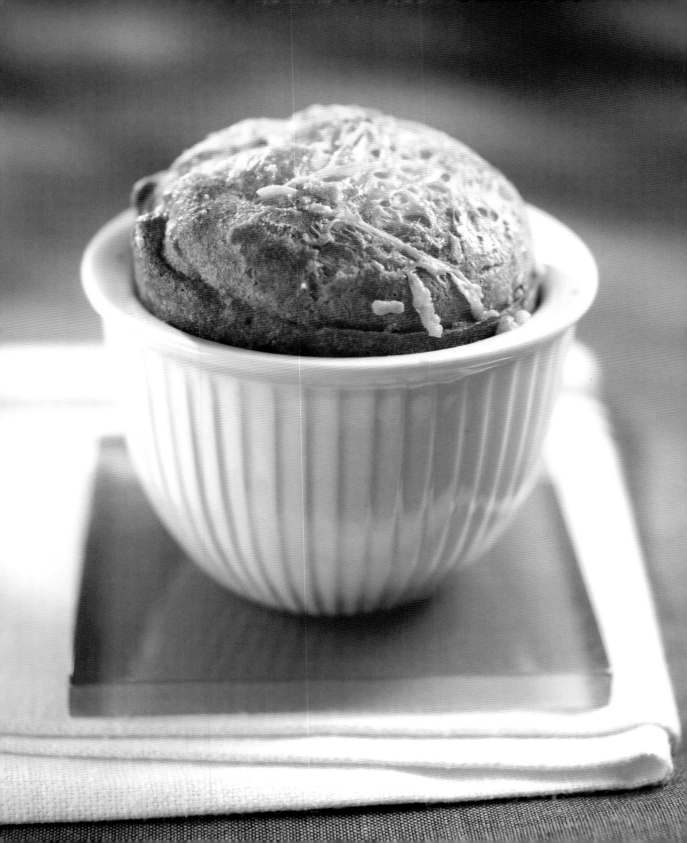

Quick Nut Bread

This is a quick bread, made without yeast. You can use other nuts instead of walnuts, and the bread may be baked in virtually anything that you can put in your oven; just remember to fill the container only three-quarters full. If you don't, it will overflow when it expands, and you'll have a big mess to clean up!

3	tablespoons sugar substitute
60 g (2 oz)	sugar
80 ml (3 fl oz)	rapeseed (canola) oil
1	egg, beaten
350 ml (12 fl oz)	skimmed milk
185 g (6½ oz)	plain flour
115 g (4 oz)	wholemeal flour
1	tablespoon baking powder
½	teaspoon bicarbonate of soda
1	teaspoon salt
115 g (4 oz)	walnuts, finely chopped

Preheat the oven to 180°C/350°F/gas 4. Coat a 23 × 13 cm (9 × 5 in or 2 lb) loaf tin with cooking spray.

In a medium bowl, thoroughly combine the sugar substitute, sugar, oil and egg. Stir in the milk. Add both flours, baking powder, bicarbonate of soda and salt, and stir until smooth. Fold in the nuts. Place the mixture into the prepared tin.

Bake for 1 hour, or until the loaf is brown on the top and firm to the touch in the centre. Cool in the tin for 15 minutes, then remove from the tin and cool on a rack. For easiest slicing, refrigerate to cool further before slicing.

Makes 16 slices

NUTRITION AT A GLANCE
Per slice: Energy 185 cals/774 kJ; 10 g fat (of which 1 g saturates), 4 g protein, 20 g carbohydrate (of which 5 g sugars), 1 g fibre, 274 mg sodium

Pancakes with Peachy Compote

This delicious combination will fast become a breakfast favourite.

Compote

1	peach, sliced, or 200 g (7 oz) drained sliced tinned peaches in juice
60 ml (2 fl oz)	orange juice
3	tablespoons sugar-free apricot jam or no-sugar-added pure fruit spread
1	teaspoon finely chopped crystallized ginger
½	teaspoon ground cinnamon
145 g (5 oz)	blackberries or blueberries

Pancakes

250 g (9 oz)	wholemeal flour
1	teaspoon bicarbonate of soda
½	teaspoon baking powder
½	teaspoon salt
1	egg + 1 egg white
480 ml (16 fl oz)	buttermilk
1	tablespoon vanilla extract
2	teaspoons rapeseed (canola) oil

To make the compote: In a small saucepan, combine the peaches, orange juice, apricot jam, ginger and cinnamon. Cook, stirring occasionally, over medium heat for 5 minutes, or until the fruit is soft. Add the berries and cook for 2 minutes longer. Keep warm over very low heat.

To make the pancakes: In a large bowl, combine the flour, bicarbonate of soda, baking powder and salt.

In a medium bowl, whisk together the egg and egg white until very foamy. Whisk in the buttermilk, vanilla extract and oil. Stir into the flour mixture just until the batter is combined.

Coat a large non-stick frying pan with cooking spray and place over medium heat. When hot, spoon 1–2 tablespoons of the batter into the pan to form a 10 cm (4 in) pancake. Cook for 2 to 3 minutes, or until the bottom is browned. Turn and cook for a further 1 to 2 minutes, or until golden brown. Transfer to a plate and keep warm. Repeat to make a total of 12 pancakes. Serve the pancakes with the warm compote.

Makes 12 pancakes

NUTRITION AT A GLANCE
Per pancake: Energy 141 cals/590 kJ; 3 g fat (of which 0.5 g saturates), 7 g protein, 23 g carbohydrate (of which 9 g sugars), 2 g fibre, 87 mg sodium

Buckwheat Pancakes

Buckwheat sounds like a grain, but it is really a summer annual. It is often planted by beekeepers, because the flower is very high in nectar.

115 g (4 oz)	buckwheat flour
125 g (4½ oz)	wholemeal flour
1	egg, beaten
1	tablespoon baking powder
480 ml (16 fl oz)	water
115 g (4 oz)	unsweetened apple sauce or purée
1	teaspoon vanilla extract

In a bowl, thoroughly combine the buckwheat flour, wholemeal flour, egg and baking powder, mixing until evenly blended. Add the water, apple sauce and vanilla extract, and stir until only small lumps remain.

Coat a large non-stick frying pan with cooking spray and place over medium heat. Working in batches, pour about 5 tablespoons of the batter into the hot pan to form a 12–15 cm (5–6 in) pancake. Cook for 2 to 3 minutes, or until the bottom is browned. Turn and cook for a further 1 to 2 minutes, or until golden brown. Transfer to a plate and keep warm. Repeat to make a total of 12 pancakes.

Makes 12 pancakes

NUTRITION AT A GLANCE
Per pancake: Energy 77 cals/322 kJ; 1 g fat (of which 0.5 g saturates), 3 g protein, 16 g carbohydrate (of which 1 g sugars), 2 g fibre, 144 mg sodium

Oat Pancakes

These pancakes have a rather dense texture. For a change of flavour, you could add a teaspoon of ground cinnamon, nutmeg, cloves or your favourite flavouring extract.

100 g (3½ oz)	rolled oats
480 ml (16 fl oz)	skimmed milk
1	egg
60 g (2 oz)	wholemeal flour
4	tablespoons toasted wheat germ
1	tablespoon baking powder
2	teaspoons sugar substitute
2	teaspoons rapeseed (canola) oil
½	teaspoon salt

In a medium bowl, combine the oats and milk and leave to stand for 10 minutes. Stir in the egg, flour, wheat germ, baking powder, sugar substitute, oil and salt, mixing until evenly blended and only small lumps remain. Let the batter stand for 30 minutes in the refrigerator.

Coat a large non-stick frying pan with cooking spray and place over medium heat. When hot, spoon 4 tablespoons of batter into the pan and spread to form a 12–15 cm (5–6 in) pancake. Cook for 3 to 4 minutes, or until the top starts to bubble and the bottom is browned. Turn and cook for a further 1 to 2 minutes, or until golden brown. Transfer to a plate and keep warm. Repeat to make a total of 12 pancakes.

Makes 12 pancakes

NUTRITION AT A GLANCE
Per pancake: Energy 100 cals/418 kJ; 4 g fat (of which 0.5 g saturates), 5 g protein, 13 g carbohydrate (of which 3 g sugars), 2 g fibre, 244 mg sodium

Ricotta Crêpes with Cherries

Kamut's appealing, nutty flavour works well in these crêpes. As an alternative, try using spelt flour, which has a similar flavour.

Crêpes

45 g (1½ oz)	kamut or spelt flour
2	tablespoons wholemeal flour
⅛	teaspoon salt
80 ml (3 fl oz)	apple juice
120 ml (4 fl oz)	water
1	large egg, lightly beaten
4	teaspoons melted trans-fat-free butter substitute

Filling

250 g (9 oz)	ricotta cheese (reduced-fat if available), or virtually fat-free fromage frais
285 g (10 oz)	pitted sweet cherries
2	tablespoons sugar-free maple syrup (optional)

To make the crêpes: In a large bowl, combine both flours and the salt. In another bowl, whisk together the apple juice, water, egg and 2 teaspoons of the melted butter substitute. Whisk into the flour mixture to make a smooth batter.

Coat a 20 cm (8 in) non-stick frying pan with cooking spray and place over medium heat. Add 1 teaspoon of the butter substitute. Pour 2 tablespoons of batter into the hot pan and quickly tilt the pan to coat the bottom with a thin layer of the batter. (If the batter seems too thick, add 1 to 2 tablespoons water.) Cook for 1 minute, or until the bottom is lightly browned. Turn and cook for a further 30 to 60 seconds. Slide the crêpe onto a plate and cover with foil to keep warm. Continue making crêpes in the same fashion, adding the remaining 1 teaspoon of butter substitute to the pan after making the second crêpe.

To make the filling and assemble: Place a crêpe on a plate, attractive side down. Arrange a quarter of the ricotta or fromage frais and a quarter of the cherries on the crêpe and fold in quarters. Repeat with the remaining ingredients. Drizzle with syrup.

Makes 4 crêpes

NUTRITION AT A GLANCE

Per crêpe: Energy 243 cals/1017 kJ; 14 g fat (of which 3 g saturates), 9 g protein, 22 g carbohydrate (of which 6 g sugars), 2 g fibre, 353 mg sodium

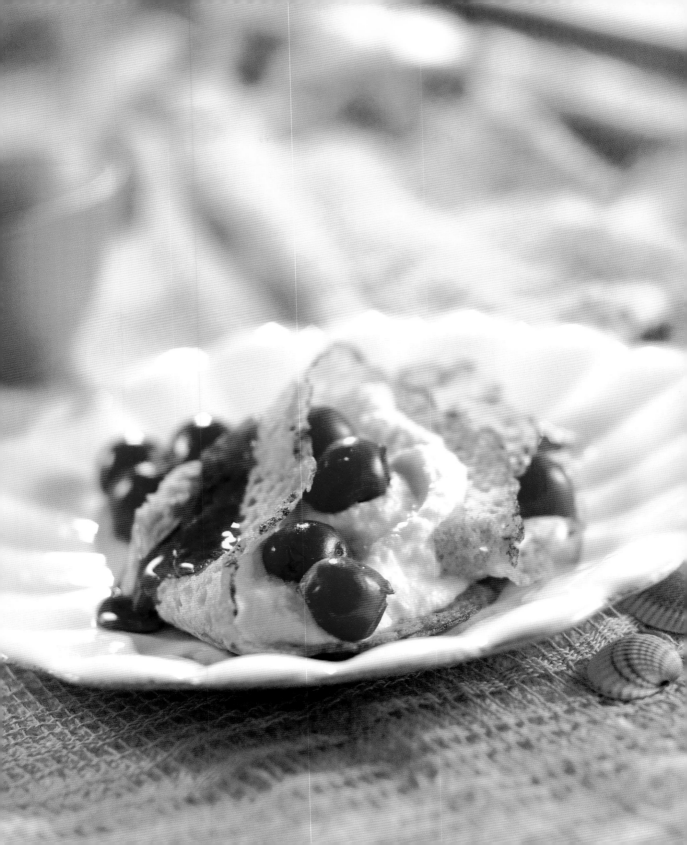

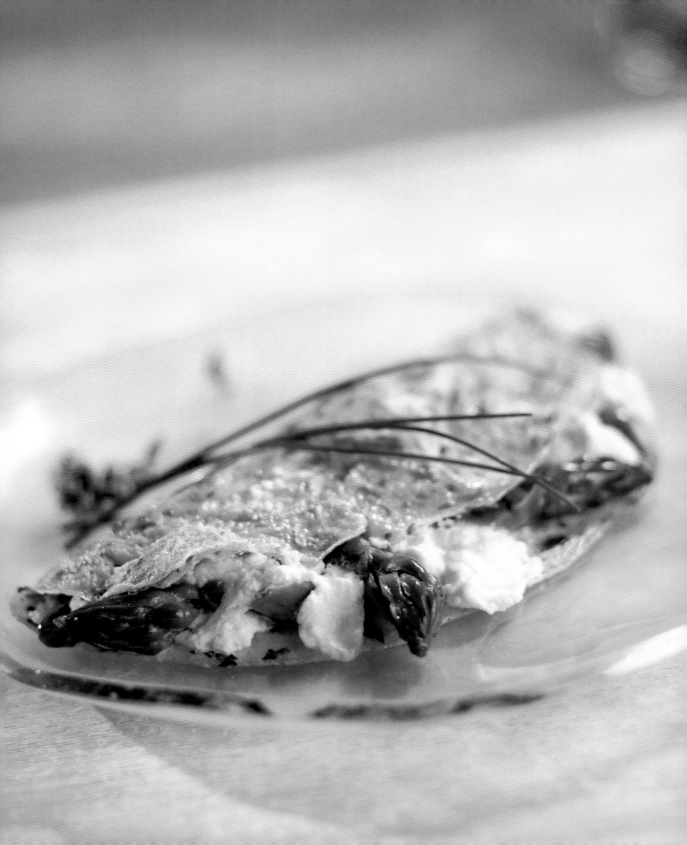

Asparagus Omelettes with Goat's Cheese

If you don't have fresh thyme, basil or dill also work very nicely.

8	eggs		⅛	teaspoon salt
60 ml (2 fl oz)	skimmed milk		230 g (8 oz)	asparagus, trimmed and cut into 2–3 cm (1 in) pieces
2	tablespoons finely chopped spring onions			
2	tablespoons chopped fresh thyme leaves		60 ml (2 fl oz)	water
			4	tablespoons crumbled goat's cheese
2	tablespoons chopped fresh parsley			fresh chives, to garnish
½	teaspoon ground black pepper			

In a medium bowl, whisk together the eggs and milk. Stir in the spring onions, thyme, parsley, pepper and salt.

Place the asparagus and water in a large microwaveable bowl. Cover with pierced plastic wrap and microwave on high power for 4 minutes, or until just tender, stirring after 2 minutes. Drain and pat dry.

Coat a 20 cm (8 in) non-stick frying pan with cooking spray and place over medium heat. When hot, pour a quarter of the egg mixture into the pan, tilting it to cover the bottom of the pan. Cook for 2 to 3 minutes, or until the bottom just begins to set, then reduce the heat to medium–low. Sprinkle with 1 tablespoon of the cheese. Add a quarter of the asparagus and cook for a further 2 to 3 minutes, or until the eggs are almost set.

Using a large spatula, fold the omelette in half over the filling and continue cooking until the omelette is golden and the cheese melted. Turn onto a plate and keep warm.

Coat the frying pan with cooking spray and repeat the process with the remaining ingredients to make 3 more omelettes. Serve hot, garnished with the chives.

Makes 4 omelettes

NUTRITION AT A GLANCE
Per omelette: Energy 206 cals/862 kJ; 14 g fat (of which 5 g saturates), 17 g protein, 2 g carbohydrate (of which 2 g sugars), 1 g fibre, 559 mg sodium

Vegetable Frittata with Parmesan

This hearty frittata is chock-full of vegetables, making for a very satisfying breakfast.

2	tablespoons trans-fat-free butter substitute
1	onion, chopped
2	courgettes (zucchini), thinly sliced
4	large mushrooms, chopped
1	red pepper (capsicum), chopped
½	teaspoon salt
¼	teaspoon dried thyme, crushed
¼	teaspoon ground black pepper
8	large eggs, at room temperature
1½	tablespoons grated Parmesan cheese (optional)

Place the grill rack in the lowest position (15–18 cm/6–7 in from the heat source) and preheat the grill.

Melt 1 tablespoon of the butter substitute in a large ovenproof non-stick frying pan over medium heat. Add the onion, courgettes, mushrooms, pepper, ¼ teaspoon of the salt, the thyme and ⅛ teaspoon of the pepper. Cook, stirring occasionally, for 8 minutes, or until the vegetables are tender and no juices remain in the pan.

In a large bowl, combine the eggs, the remaining ¼ teaspoon salt and ⅛ teaspoon pepper and the cheese, if using.

Melt the remaining 1 tablespoon butter substitute in the frying pan with the vegetables over very low heat. Pour in the egg mixture. Cook, uncovered and without stirring, for 15 minutes, or until only the top remains runny. Place the frying pan under the grill and cook for 2 minutes, or until the eggs are just set. Slide the frittata onto a large serving plate.

Makes 4 servings

NUTRITION AT A GLANCE
Per serving: Energy 254 cals/1063 kJ; 19 g fat (of which 5 g saturates), 16 g protein, 5 g carbohydrate (of which 4 g sugars), 1.5 g fibre, 549 mg sodium

MY SOUTH BEACH DIET

WE COULD EAT THIS WAY FOR THE REST OF OUR LIVES.

Our only daughter left for college last year, and my husband, Jack, and I were dealing with 'empty nest' feelings, not to mention the added stress of turning 50! Major turning points like these get you thinking about the future. We both gained weight in our forties, and have family histories of heart disease. When the cardiologist said that Jack's high cholesterol readings should be a wake-up call, we knew we had to get serious about making changes.

I picked up the South Beach Diet book after hearing about it in *Prevention* magazine. What really caught my attention was the clear description of the connections between cholesterol, diet and heart health.

We decided that we were ready to tackle this new preventive lifestyle change together. Jack has always been a morning-coffee-and-pastry guy, not a big egg eater, so finding breakfasts that he enjoyed was tough those first weeks. Learning the basic foods to avoid from the start was really helpful. When I missed my potatoes, I tried Surprise South Beach 'Mashed Potatoes', made with cauliflower, and loved them!

After the first two weeks (Phase 1), my husband lost 3.5 kg (8 lb), and I lost 2.5 kg (6 lb). It wasn't as much as we'd hoped, but we both had much more energy in the summer evenings for walks or even a round of golf after work. We planned our meals together and found ourselves eating out less. When we do go out, we've been choosing restaurants that serve Mediterranean food – hummus, couscous, grilled fish, meats and vegetables. Or we focus on trying new salads, and choose main dishes to share.

Jack struggled to stay on the plan while travelling for work – that was probably the hardest challenge. Funny coincidence, he sat next to a woman on a plane who mentioned that it was the first time she didn't need a seatbelt extender, thanks to a new diet. Turns out she'd been on the South Beach Diet, too!

Early success really convinced us to stay with the plan. Jack has now lost 7 kg (over a stone), and I've lost 5 kg (11 lb). Jack's cholesterol check-up is next month, and we're expecting an improvement. The boost in energy and minimal cravings for old familiar foods made it clear that we could eat this way for the rest of our lives. We can't wait to see our daughter's face when she returns home for the holidays! – *CYNTHIA AND JACK C.*

Smoked Ham 'Soufflé'

This mock soufflé is easy to make; once you've assembled it, just pop it in the oven while you get on with something else.

2	eggs
4	egg whites
350 ml (12 fl oz)	skimmed milk
170 g (6 oz)	reduced-fat mature Cheddar cheese, grated
4	slices wholemeal bread, cubed
115 g (4 oz)	mushrooms, sliced
90 g (3 oz)	broccoli florets or 4–6 asparagus spears, trimmed and chopped
115 g (4 oz)	lean smoked ham, chopped
½	teaspoon Italian herb seasoning

Preheat the oven to 180°C/350°F/gas 4. Coat a 2-litre (3½-pint) baking dish with cooking spray.

In a large bowl, beat the eggs and egg whites until frothy. Stir in the milk, cheese, bread, mushrooms, broccoli or asparagus, ham and herb seasoning. Pour into the prepared baking dish.

Bake for 40 to 45 minutes, or until golden and a knife inserted in the centre comes out clean. Serve hot.

Makes 4 servings

NUTRITION AT A GLANCE
Per serving: Energy 305 cals/1276 kJ; 12 g fat (of which 6 g saturates), 30 g protein, 20 g carbohydrate (of which 5 g sugars), 3 g fibre, 958 mg sodium

Sausage and Cheese Breakfast Cups

These egg 'muffins' make a hearty breakfast that can be eaten on the run.
Make them ahead and warm them in the microwave for a quick breakfast treat.

115 g (4 oz)	turkey sausage, crumbled, or turkey bacon or lean bacon, finely chopped
½	green pepper (capsicum), finely chopped
170 g (6 oz)	mushrooms, sliced
¼	onion, finely chopped
4	large eggs, beaten
60 g (2 oz)	reduced-fat Cheddar cheese, grated

Preheat the oven to 180°C/350°F/gas 4. Coat a 6-cup non-stick muffin tin with cooking spray or line with paper cake cases.

Coat a non-stick frying pan with cooking spray and place over medium-high heat. Add the sausage, pepper and onion and cook for 5 minutes, or until the sausage is no longer pink. Spoon the mixture into a bowl and cool slightly. Add the mushrooms to the pan and cook until just tender, then add to the bowl. Stir in the eggs.

Divide the mixture among the prepared muffin cups. Sprinkle with the cheese, then bake for 20 minutes, or until the egg is set.

Makes 6 cups

NUTRITION AT A GLANCE
Per serving: Energy 112 cals/469 kJ; 7 g fat (of which 2.5 g saturates), 12 g protein, 1 g carbohydrate (of which 1 g sugars), 0.5 g fibre, 474 mg sodium

Quiche with Swiss Cheese and Fennel

The distinctive personalities of fennel and Swiss cheese are made for each other. Enjoy this dish for breakfast or brunch, or as a first course when making dinner for friends.

Crust

145 g (5 oz)	wholemeal flour
¼	teaspoon salt
2	tablespoons rapeseed (canola) oil
2	tablespoons trans-fat-free butter substitute, cold and cut into small pieces
2–3	tablespoons iced water

Filling

90 g (3 oz)	fennel bulb, thinly sliced
6	spring onions, chopped
3	eggs
150 ml (5 fl oz)	evaporated milk (low-fat if available)
150 ml (5 fl oz)	skimmed milk
1½	teaspoons Dijon mustard
¼	teaspoon ground nutmeg
¼	teaspoon ground black pepper
60 g (2 oz)	reduced-fat Swiss-style cheese, grated
1	tablespoon grated Parmesan cheese
	pinch of paprika

To make the crust: Preheat the oven to 220°C/425°F/gas 7. Coat a 23 cm (9 in) tart tin with cooking spray.

In a large bowl or food processor, combine the flour and salt. Blend with a pastry blender or process briefly to mix. Add the oil and butter substitute and stir or process until the mixture resembles fine breadcrumbs. While stirring constantly or with the motor of the food processor running, add the water, 1 tablespoon at a time, and stir or process for 30 seconds, or until the pastry barely comes together. Transfer to a work surface and pat the pastry into a flattened disk.

Place the pastry between 2 sheets of greaseproof paper and roll out to a 28 cm (11 in) circle. Remove the top sheet and invert the pastry into the prepared tart tin. Remove the remaining sheet of greaseproof paper and fit the pastry into the tin. Use a fork to prick holes in the bottom and sides of the pastry. Line with a piece of foil and top it with a layer of pie weights or dried beans or rice.

Bake for 10 minutes. Remove the weights and foil and bake for a further 4 minutes, or until the pastry is dry but has not begun to brown.

To make the filling: Coat a non-stick frying pan with cooking spray and place over medium heat. Add the sliced fennel and cook for 5 minutes, or until soft. Add the spring onions and cook for 2 minutes.

In a medium bowl, whisk together the eggs, evaporated milk, skimmed milk, mustard, nutmeg and pepper.

Sprinkle the fennel mixture over the bottom of the baked pastry shell and top with the Swiss cheese. Pour in the egg mixture and sprinkle the top with the Parmesan and paprika.

Bake for 30 minutes, or until a knife inserted in the centre comes out clean. Cool on a rack for 10 minutes.

Makes 6 servings

NUTRITION AT A GLANCE
Per serving: Energy 274 cals/1147 kJ; 15 g fat (of which 5 g saturates), 14 g protein, 21 g carbohydrate (of which 4 g sugars), 2 g fibre, 413 mg sodium

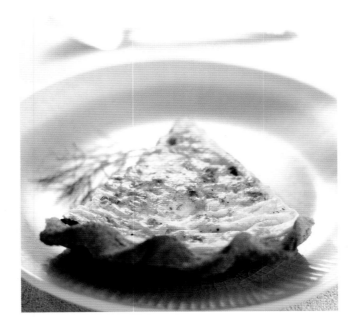

Hot Scrambled Tofu

Tabasco adds a fiery kick to tofu.

570 g (1 lb 4 oz)	silken tofu
2	tablespoons extra virgin olive oil
4	spring onions, white part only, finely chopped
¼	tablespoon turmeric
	salt
	freshly ground black pepper
	Tabasco
60 g (2 oz)	reduced-fat cheese, grated
¼	teaspoon paprika

Cover a large baking sheet with paper towels. Place the tofu on the towels in a single layer. Cover with more paper towels and pat down until dry. Discard the paper towels. Crumble the tofu.

Heat the oil in a large frying pan over medium–high heat. Add the spring onions and cook, stirring frequently, for 3 minutes, or until soft. Stir in the tofu and turmeric. Add salt, pepper and Tabasco to taste. Cook for 2 minutes, or until the tofu is firm.

Divide among 4 serving plates. Sprinkle with the cheese and paprika and serve hot.

Makes 4 servings

NUTRITION AT A GLANCE

Per serving: Energy 195 cals/816 kJ; 14 g fat (of which 3 g saturates), 16 g protein, 1 g carbohydrate (of which 0.5 g sugars), 0 g fibre, 593 mg sodium

Breakfast Croque Monsieur

Why not have this classic French ham and cheese sandwich for breakfast in Phases 2 and 3?

8	slices wholemeal bread, crusts removed
4	tablespoons trans-fat-free butter substitute, melted
115 g (4 oz)	reduced-fat mozzarella cheese, thinly sliced
170 g (6 oz)	boiled ham, thinly sliced

Brush 1 side of each slice of bread with the butter substitute and top with slices of cheese. Add the ham and cover with the remaining bread, dry side up.

Generously brush a large unheated frying pan with butter substitute. Working in batches if necessary, add the sandwiches and cook over medium heat for 4 minutes, or until lightly browned on the bottom. Turn the sandwiches over and rebrush the frying pan with butter substitute. Cover and cook for 4 minutes, or until the cheese is melted and the bread is browned. Serve immediately.

Makes 4 sandwiches

NUTRITION AT A GLANCE
Per sandwich: Energy 350 cals/1465 kJ; 18 g fat (of which 5 g saturates), 20 g protein, 24 g carbohydrate (of which 1 g sugars), 3 g fibre, 1179 mg sodium

Turkey Patties with Fennel

These tasty sausage patties are fragrant with fennel seed. If you like, you can substitute 2 tablespoons wholemeal breadcrumbs for the chopped nuts to make this a Phase 2 recipe.

455 g (1 lb)	turkey breast, minced
¼	onion, grated
1	egg, beaten
2	tablespoons finely chopped pecan nuts
¼	teaspoon fennel seeds, finely crushed

In a bowl, combine the turkey, onion, egg, nuts and fennel seeds. Shape the mixture into 8 patties.

Coat a large non-stick frying pan with cooking spray and place over medium heat for 1 minute. Working in batches if necessary, add the patties and cook for 5 minutes on each side, or until a thermometer inserted in the centre of a patty registers 75°C/165°F and the meat is no longer pink.

Makes 8 patties

NUTRITION AT A GLANCE
Per patty: Energy 104 cals/435 kJ; 4 g fat (of which 0.5 g saturates), 15 g protein, 1 g carbohydrate (of which 0.5 g sugars), 0.5 g fibre, 33 mg sodium

Apricot-Glazed Bacon

Ten minutes is all it takes to make this breakfast treat.

455 g (1 lb)	lean bacon, in 5 mm (¼ in) thick rashers
4	tablespoons sugar-free apricot jam or no-sugar-added pure fruit spread
¼	teaspoon mustard powder

Preheat the grill.

Place the bacon on a grill rack 8 cm (3 in) from the heat and cook for 4 minutes.

Meanwhile, in a small bowl, mix together the jam and mustard. Turn the bacon and brush with the jam mixture. Grill for a further 4 minutes, or until the bacon is well done.

Makes 4 servings

NUTRITION AT A GLANCE
Per serving: Energy 190 cals/795 kJ; 8 g fat (of which 3 g saturates), 23 g protein, 8 g carbohydrate (of which 8 g sugars), 0 g fibre, 2154 mg sodium

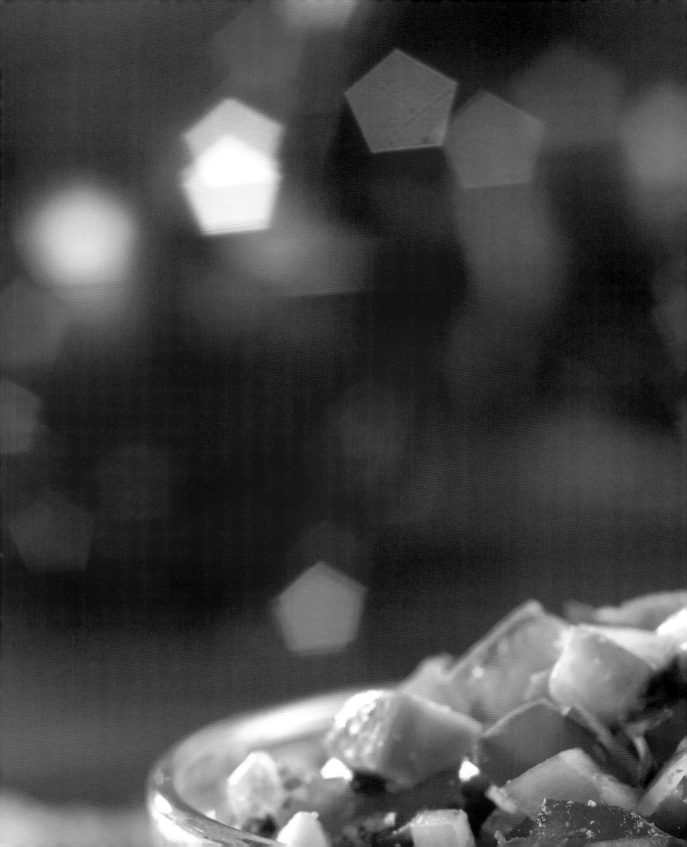

STARTERS AND SNACKS

SNACKS ARE AN EXTREMELY IMPORTANT COMPONENT OF THE SOUTH BEACH DIET. TWO OF THE MOST DANGEROUS TIMES IN A DIETER'S DAY ARE THE HOURS BETWEEN BREAKFAST AND LUNCH — THE COFFEE BREAK WITH A BISCUIT — AND THEN THAT POINT IN MID-AFTERNOON WHEN YOUR ENERGY BEGINS TO FLAG, AND YOU REACH FOR A PICK-ME-UP IN THE FORM OF A CAKE OR CHOCOLATE. NOTHING UNDERMINES SELF-CONTROL LIKE THE COMBINATION OF HUNGER AND WEARINESS, AND NEXT THING YOU KNOW, YOU'VE UNDONE ALL YOUR GOOD EFFORTS THE REST OF THE DAY. THIS IS WHY WE DECIDED THAT THIS EATING PLAN WOULD ALLOW YOU AT LEAST TWO SNACKS DAILY.

THESE SNACKS ARE HEALTHY COMBINATIONS OF PROTEIN, GOOD FATS AND GOOD CARBS THAT WILL SATISFY BETWEEN-MEAL CRAVINGS WITHOUT FILLING YOU UP WITH BAD CARBS. WE'VE ALSO PUT TOGETHER A SELECTION OF FIRST COURSES THAT WILL SEND THE RIGHT MESSAGE TO THE APPETITE CENTRE IN YOUR BRAIN. YOU'LL MAKE THESE DISHES AGAIN AND AGAIN.

Spicy Prawns in Lettuce Wraps

This impressive starter wraps hot-and-spicy prawns in cool-and-crisp lettuce.
Save any leftovers for a light yet satisfying lunch the next day.

1	tablespoon groundnut (peanut) oil
455 g (1 lb)	large uncooked prawns, peeled, de-veined and coarsely chopped
60 g (2 oz)	celery, finely chopped
5	water chestnuts, chopped
1	clove garlic, finely chopped
1	teaspoon finely chopped fresh ginger
1	tablespoon hoisin sauce
1	tablespoon light soy sauce
1	tablespoon rice wine vinegar
8	large lettuce leaves
	toasted chopped peanuts, to garnish

Heat the oil in a wok or large non-stick frying pan over medium-high heat. Add the prawns and stir-fry until they are opaque. Transfer the prawns to a bowl and set aside.

Add the celery, water chestnuts, garlic and ginger, and stir-fry until the vegetables are crisp-tender.

Return the prawns to the wok and add the hoisin sauce, soy sauce and vinegar. Cook for 1 minute, or until heated through.

Divide the mixture evenly among the lettuce leaves. Sprinkle with the peanuts.

Makes 4 servings

NUTRITION AT A GLANCE
Per serving: Energy 189 cals/790 kJ; 7 g fat (of which 1.5 g saturates), 28 g protein, 2 g carbohydrate (of which 1 g sugars), 1 g fibre, 500 mg sodium

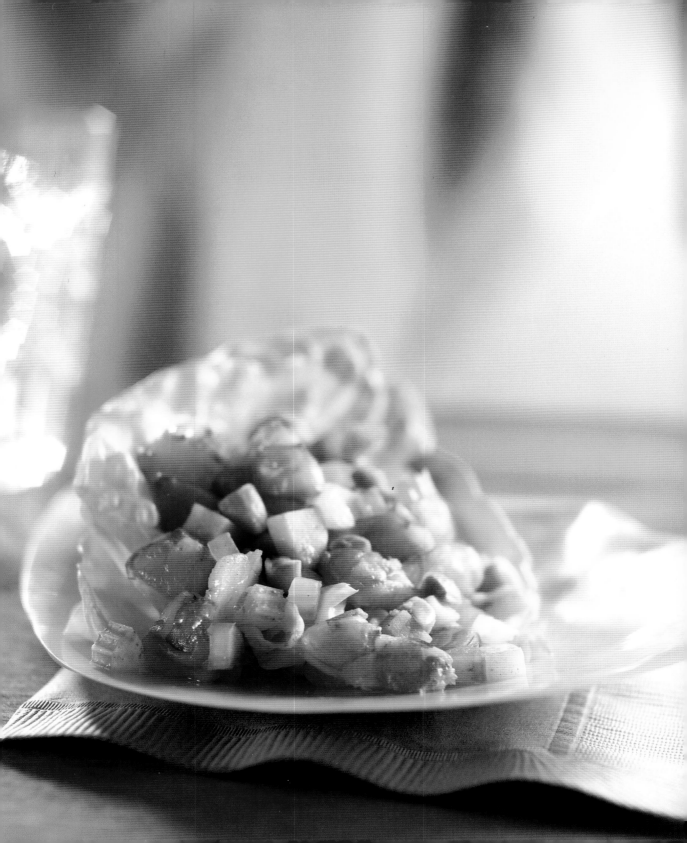

From the Menu of . . .

PASHA'S

900 Lincoln Road, Miami Beach, Florida

CHEFS TULIN TUZEL AND CARLA ELLEK

Pasha's serves healthy and delicious Mediterranean food, proving once again the two are never mutually exclusive.

Artichokes in Olive Oil

PHASE 1

4 globe artichokes, trimmed down to the hearts	juice of 1 lemon
8 spring onions, cut into 2 cm (1 in) pieces	120 ml (4 fl oz) water
1 medium onion, sliced	2 teaspoons salt
4 teaspoons extra virgin olive oil	6 tablespoons chopped fresh dill
1 lemon, sliced	lemon wedges, to garnish

Place the artichokes in a saucepan with the spring onions, onion, oil, lemon, lemon juice and water. Cover and cook over low heat for 35 minutes.

Add the salt and most of the dill, reserving some dill for garnish. Baste the artichokes and continue to cook for 20 minutes, or until tender.

Leave to cool, then sprinkle with the remaining dill. Serve cold, with wedges of lemon to garnish.

Makes 4 servings

NUTRITION AT A GLANCE

Per serving: Energy 144 cals/602kJ; 12 g fat (of which 2 g saturates), 4 g protein, 6 g carbohydrate (of which 5 g sugars), 3 g fibre, 1169 mg sodium

Grilled Tempeh Triangles

Tempeh is a soya-based protein that's frequently enjoyed by vegetarians as a meat alternative. You can serve these triangles as a first course or with steamed or stir-fried vegetables as a main dish.

455 g (1 lb)	tempeh, cut into triangles
1	tablespoon groundnut (peanut) oil
½	teaspoon toasted sesame oil
1	teaspoon grated fresh ginger
2	tablespoons light soy sauce
1	teaspoon finely chopped garlic
2	tablespoons sliced spring onions, to garnish

Place the tempeh in a shallow glass dish. In a small bowl, mix the peanut oil, sesame oil, ginger, soy sauce and garlic. Pour the mixture over the tempeh, turning the pieces to coat well. Place in the refrigerator for 4 hours or overnight.

Preheat the grill to medium-high. Place a large piece of foil on the grill. Place the tempeh triangles on the foil and grill for 3 to 4 minutes on each side, until golden brown. Sprinkle the tempeh with spring onions and serve hot.

Makes 4 servings

NUTRITION AT A GLANCE
Per serving: Energy 180 cals/753 kJ; 12 g fat (of which 2 g saturates), 10 g protein, 13 g carbohydrate (of which 7 g sugars), 1 g fibre, 450 mg sodium

From the Menu of . . .

CASA TUA RESTAURANT

1700 James Avenue, Miami Beach, Florida

CHEF SERGIO SIGALA

Casa Tua is a beautiful restaurant in a converted European-style villa. This fabulous Tuna Tartare is Phase 3 with bread but Phase 1 if served with cucumber instead.

Casa Tua Tuna Tartare

PHASE 1

455 g (1 lb) fresh, top-quality (sushi-grade) tuna, chopped

15 g (½ oz) capers in salt, rinsed and drained

90 g (3 oz) small black olives, pitted and chopped

60 g (2 oz) sun-dried tomatoes, chopped

1 tablespoon chopped fresh coriander

½ tablespoon chopped fresh red chilli (wear rubber gloves when handling)

4 tablespoons extra virgin olive oil

1 tablespoon balsamic vinegar

½ tablespoon salt flakes

Mix the tuna, capers, olives, tomatoes, coriander and chilli, and season with the olive oil, vinegar and salt flakes.

Note: if you like, serve with cucumber slices or – on Phase 3 only – with grilled or toasted French bread.

Makes 4 servings

NUTRITION AT A GLANCE
Per serving: Energy 262 cals/1096 kJ; 16 g fat (of which 2.5 g saturates), 27 g protein, 2 g carbohydrate (of which 2 g sugars), 1 g fibre, 1193 mg sodium

Grilled Clams Gremolata

Gremolata is a mixture of finely chopped parsley, garlic and lemon zest. It adds a fresh, light flavour when sprinkled over seafood.

3 tablespoons chopped fresh parsley

2 cloves garlic, finely chopped

½ teaspoon grated lemon zest

24 fresh clams, scrubbed

Tabasco (optional)

Preheat the grill or barbecue.

In a small cup, combine the parsley, garlic and lemon zest.

Place the clams on a baking sheet and grill or cook over medium-hot coals for 5 minutes, or until the shells open. Discard any unopened clams. Sprinkle the parsley mixture over the clams and serve hot. Serve with Tabasco, if using.

Makes 4 servings

NUTRITION AT A GLANCE

Per serving: Energy 58 cals/242 kJ; 1 g fat (of which 0.5 g saturates), 11 g protein, 0.5 g carbohydrate (of which 0 g sugars), 0 g fibre, 131 mg sodium

Entertaining, South Beach-Style

Planning a party menu around a weight loss regime may not seem like the most festive thing you'll ever do. But as Miami's top chefs have demonstrated – for example in the chefs' recipes sprinkled throughout this book – South Beach-legal dishes can be done in high culinary style. The diet offers lots of options for food to serve while entertaining at home, too.

We discussed this with party planner Susan Kleinberg, who came up with several ways to accommodate the diet at social events. If you're having a drinks party, you'll probably want finger food. Serve fresh vegetables, either raw or grilled with olive oil, with a low-fat or fat-free dip. Bowls of cashews or other nuts are a party staple. Try prawns – poached, steamed or grilled. Smoked salmon with reduced-fat cream cheese on a wholegrain cracker or pumpernickel square is another favourite. You can push the boat out with caviar and still be well within the guidelines.

If you're serving a buffet dinner, you'll want two or three main dishes to choose from. A seared tuna fillet or a grilled salmon are great choices. Both can be prepared ahead of time and served at room temperature. Another good choice is roasted turkey breast or chicken breast in a Dijon mustard sauce. You can serve marinated steak for red-meat fans. All of these main courses are fine on the South Beach Diet.

For side dishes, you can set up a salad bar with marinated vegetables, mixed salad leaves, and various optional extras, such as reduced-fat cheeses, fruit and nuts. In place of the usual salad carbs such as croutons or pasta, offer salad made with tabbouleh, bulgur wheat, or barley. You can even have wholewheat pitta bread with hummus on the side.

For dessert, you can create a beautiful berry bar, offering strawberries, blueberries, or whatever else is in season, accompanied by a bowl of shaved dark chocolate. Or you might serve melted dark chocolate and large strawberries on skewers for dipping. A dollop of whipped cream doesn't seem completely out of order, considering how virtuous you've been with the rest of the party menu.

Salmon Bites

This satisfying snack is simple to prepare and makes a great party appetizer.

230 g (8 oz)	reduced-fat cream cheese
400 g (14 oz)	tinned salmon, drained and flaked, skin and bones removed
1	tablespoon finely chopped onion
1	tablespoon lemon juice
1	teaspoon prepared horseradish
¼	teaspoon salt
¼	teaspoon liquid smoke (optional)
60 g (2 oz)	finely chopped almonds
4	tablespoons finely chopped fresh parsley

In a large bowl, beat the cream cheese to soften it, then add the salmon, onion, lemon juice, horseradish, salt and liquid smoke, if using; mix thoroughly. Refrigerate for 4 hours, or until firm.

In a small bowl, combine the almonds and parsley. Shape the salmon mixture into 32 balls, then roll in the almond mixture. Serve chilled.

Makes 16 servings

NUTRITION AT A GLANCE

Per serving: Energy 87 cals/364 kJ; 6 g fat (of which 2 g saturates), 8 g protein, 1 g carbohydrate (of which 0.5 g sugars), 0 g fibre, 211 mg sodium

Sun-Dried Tomato Tartlets with Cheese

Widely used in Greek cuisine, filo is a thin, delicate pastry that becomes light and flaky when baked. You can buy it fresh or frozen, from delicatessens or supermarkets. The frozen variety keeps for up to a year in the freezer.

8	sheets 43 × 28 cm (17 × 11 in) frozen filo pastry, thawed if frozen
170 g (6 oz)	ricotta cheese (reduced-fat if available)
3	tablespoons crumbled goat's cheese or feta cheese
1	egg white
1	spring onion, chopped
2	tablespoons chopped fresh basil
2	cloves garlic, finely chopped
45 g (1½ oz)	oil-packed sun-dried tomatoes, drained and chopped
	sprigs of basil, to garnish

Preheat the oven to 190°C/375°F/gas 5. Coat 24 tartlet tins (5 cm/2 in diameter), with cooking spray.

Place 1 sheet of filo pastry on a work surface. Coat with cooking spray. Top with 3 more sheets, coating each sheet with cooking spray. Cut the sheets in thirds lengthwise and then in quarters crosswise to make 12 squares. Press each square into a tartlet tin to form a shell with jagged edges. Repeat with the remaining sheets to line the remaining tartlet tins.

Bake for 5 minutes, or until golden.

Meanwhile, in a food processor, combine the ricotta, goat's cheese or feta cheese and egg white. Process until smooth. Add the spring onion, basil, garlic and tomatoes. Pulse briefly to mix. Spoon into the filo pastry shells. Bake for 5 minutes, or until lightly puffed and heated through. Garnish with basil sprigs.

Makes 24 tartlets

NUTRITION AT A GLANCE

Per 3 tartlets: Energy 145 cals/606 kJ; 6 g fat (of which 3 g saturates), 6 g protein, 19 g carbohydrate (of which 2 g sugars), 1 g fibre, 166 mg sodium

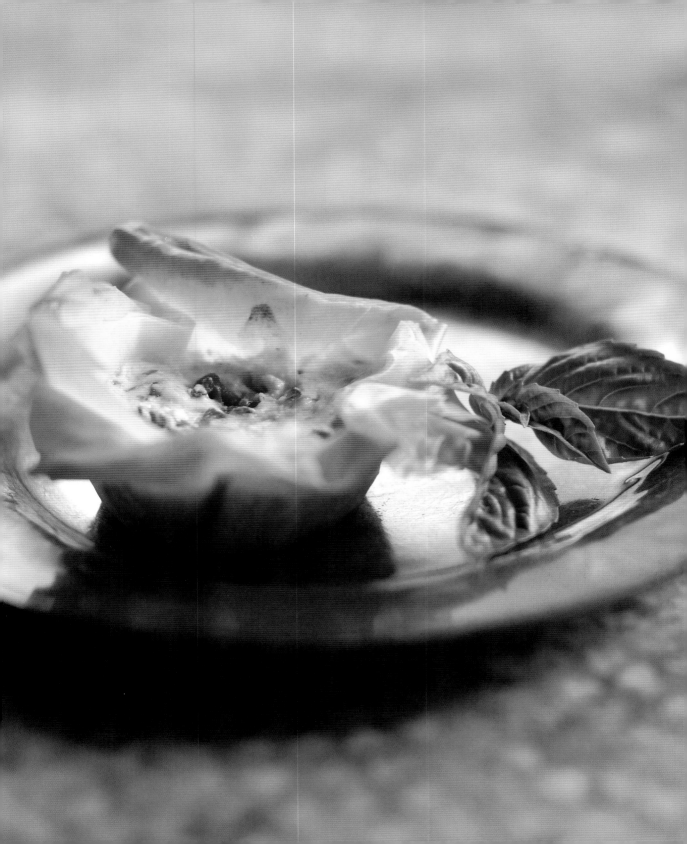

Baked Tomatoes with Crab

Fresh crabmeat on juicy ripe tomatoes makes a luscious combination. These elegant treats are easy to make and bake in just 15 minutes.

40 g (1¼ oz)	finely ground nuts, such as pecans or walnuts
2	large tomatoes, halved
125 g (4½ oz)	fresh crabmeat
115 g (4 oz)	reduced-fat Cheddar cheese, grated
60 g (2 oz)	black olives, finely chopped
30 g (1 oz)	mushrooms, finely chopped
30 g (1 oz)	parsley, finely chopped
1	clove garlic, finely chopped
½	teaspoon dried oregano
½	teaspoon dried basil

Preheat the oven to 180°C/350°F/gas 4. Coat a baking sheet with cooking spray.

Place the ground nuts on a plate. Coat the tomato halves with cooking spray. Dip the cut sides into the nuts to coat well. Place the tomatoes, cut side up, on the prepared baking sheet.

In a large bowl, combine the crabmeat, cheese, olives, mushrooms, parsley, garlic, oregano and basil. Divide the crab mixture among the tomatoes.

Bake for 15 minutes, or until hot and bubbly. Serve immediately.

Makes 4 servings

NUTRITION AT A GLANCE
Per serving: Energy 210 cals/879 kJ; 15 g fat (of which 4 g saturates), 18 g protein, 2 g carbohydrate (of which 2 g sugars), 1 g fibre, 651 mg sodium

Spiced Pickled Eggs

Planning a picnic? A long car ride? A summer day in the garden? Or maybe you just want something to go in your salad. For all those occasions and more, these eggs may just be what you're looking for.

12	large eggs
450 ml (15 fl oz)	white vinegar
1	onion, sliced and separated into rings
2	tablespoons sugar substitute
1½	teaspoons pickling spice
1	teaspoon salt

Carefully place the eggs in a large saucepan. Fill the pan with water until the eggs are covered with about 2–3 cm (1 in) of extra water. Bring the water to the boil over high heat. Turn off the heat. Cover and leave to stand for 18 minutes. Run cold water into the saucepan until all the water is cool. Remove the eggs from the pan and refrigerate until cool.

Peel the eggs, place loosely in a large pickling jar and set aside.

In a large saucepan, combine the vinegar, onion, sugar substitute, pickling spice and salt. Bring to the boil over high heat. Reduce the heat to low and simmer for 5 minutes. Pour the hot mixture over the eggs, then seal with an airtight lid. Refrigerate until ready to serve.

Makes 12 eggs

NUTRITION AT A GLANCE
Per egg: Energy 78 cals/326 kJ; 5 g fat (of which 1.5 g saturates), 6 g protein, 1 g carbohydrate (of which 0.5 g sugars), 0 g fibre, 265 mg sodium

Cottage Cheese-Stuffed Celery

This is spicy, sharp, snappy and smooth all in one bite.

115 g (4 oz)	reduced-fat cottage cheese or fromage frais
1	spring onion, finely chopped
⅛	teaspoon prepared horseradish
⅛	teaspoon Worcestershire sauce
	pinch of garlic powder
4	sticks of celery, cut into 8 cm (3 in) pieces
	paprika, to garnish

In a small bowl, combine the cheese, spring onion, horseradish, Worcestershire sauce and garlic; mix thoroughly. Spoon into the hollow side of the celery sticks and sprinkle with the paprika.

Makes 4 servings

NUTRITION AT A GLANCE

Per serving: Energy 20 cals/84 kJ; trace fat (of which 0 g saturates), 2.5 g protein, 2.5 g carbohydrate (of which 2 g sugars), 0.5 g fibre, 56 mg sodium

Reuben Wrap

You will have to have a 'rye' sense of humour for this version of the classic American Reuben sandwich; you won't find any bread in our wrap!

- 1 cabbage leaf
- 1 slice reduced-fat Swiss cheese or soya 'cheese'
- 1 slice pastrami
- 1 tablespoon coarse-grain mustard or sugar-free Thousand Island dressing
- 2 tablespoons sauerkraut

Fan the cabbage leaf on a plate. Place the cheese on the cabbage leaf and top with the pastrami. Spread the mustard or dressing onto the pastrami. Add the sauerkraut. Roll up and secure with a cocktail stick.

Makes 1 wrap

NUTRITION AT A GLANCE

Per wrap: Energy 134 cals/560 kJ; 6 g fat (of which 2.5 g saturates), 15 g protein, 6 g carbohydrate (of which 5 g sugars), 2 g fibre, 782 mg sodium

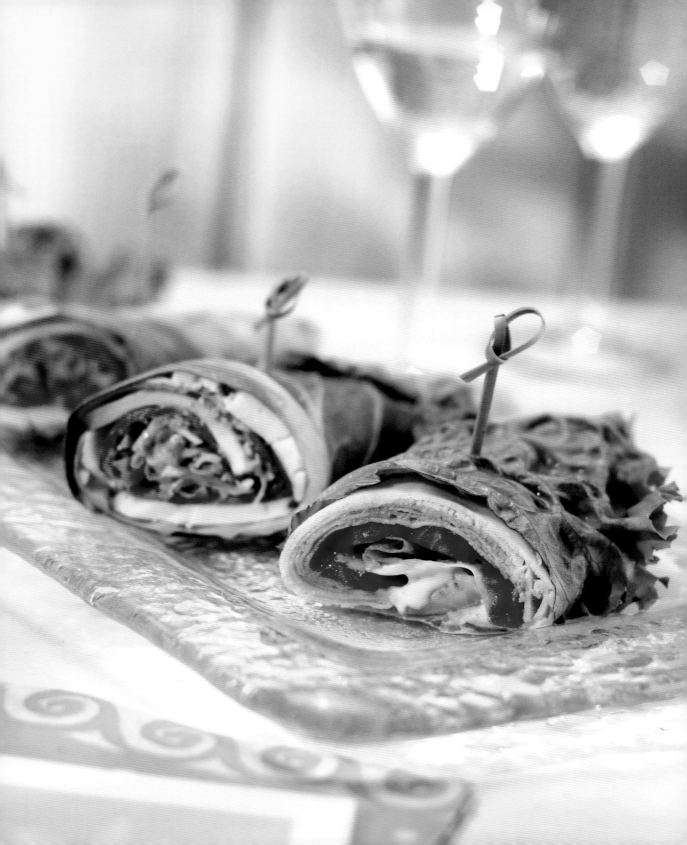

California Wrap

This is a great portable snack. Prepare it the night before and wrap it tightly in plastic wrap to keep it fresh for the next day.

1 red or green lettuce leaf

1 slice turkey breast

1 slice ham

1 thin slice tomato

1 thin slice avocado

1 teaspoon lime juice

1 leaf watercress or rocket

2 teaspoons mayonnaise

1 teaspoon rapeseed (canola) oil

Fan the lettuce leaf on a plate. Top with the turkey, ham and tomato.

In a small bowl, combine the avocado and lime juice, then place on the tomato. Top with the watercress or rocket. Mix the mayonnaise and oil together and spoon onto the watercress or rocket leaf. Roll up and secure with a cocktail stick.

Makes 1 wrap

NUTRITION AT A GLANCE

Per wrap: Energy 200 cals/837 kJ; 17 g fat (of which 3 g saturates), 10 g protein, 1 g carbohydrate (of which 1 g sugars), 0.5 g fibre, 329 mg sodium

Cheese and Turkey Roll-Ups with Nut Butter

For a Phase 2 snack, you can add the optional apple slices to these roll-ups.

4	thin slices Emmental, Port Salut or soya 'cheese', at room temperature
60 g (2 oz)	thinly sliced turkey breast
½	large apple, peeled and thinly sliced (optional for Phase 2)
1	tablespoon macadamia nut butter or 2 teaspoons unsweetened peanut butter

Place the cheese on a cutting board. Place the turkey on top. Add the apples, if using. Drizzle or spread with the macadamia nut butter or peanut butter and roll up. Secure with cocktail sticks.

Makes 4 roll-ups

NUTRITION AT A GLANCE

Per roll-up: Energy 139 cals/582 kJ; 10 g fat (of which 5 g saturates), 11 g protein, 2 g carbohydrate (of which 1.5 g sugars), 0.5 g fibre, 159 mg sodium

Peanut Dip

If you want a little something to go with your raw vegetables, this is just what you've been looking for.

250 g (9 oz)	unsalted roasted peanuts
115 g (4 oz)	fat-free natural yogurt
¼	teaspoon finely grated lemon zest
	salt

In a blender or food processor, combine the peanuts, yogurt, lemon zest and salt to taste, and process until smooth.

Makes 600 ml (20 fl oz)

NUTRITION AT A GLANCE

Per tablespoon: Energy 74 cals/310 kJ; 6 g fat (of which 1 g saturates), 4 g protein, 2 g carbohydrate (of which 1 g sugars), 1 g fibre, 63 mg sodium

Hot Ham Roll-Ups

Feel free to substitute any sugar-free jam in this recipe, and if you want to add a little lettuce, go right ahead.

8 slices baked ham

8 tablespoons sugar-free cherry jam or no-sugar-added pure fruit spread

Preheat the oven to 190°C/375°F/gas 5.

Roll the ham slices and place in a shallow baking dish. Bake for 5 minutes, or until heated through.

Place the jam in a microwaveable dish, cover and microwave on medium for 30 seconds. Stir the jam and if it is not hot enough, cover and microwave for a further 15 seconds.

Place 2 ham rolls on each of 4 serving plates. Drizzle each serving with the hot jam.

Makes 8 roll-ups

NUTRITION AT A GLANCE
Per 2 roll-ups: Energy 165 cals/690 kJ; 3 g fat (of which 1 g saturates), 11 g protein, 24 g carbohydrate (of which 23 g sugars), 0 g fibre, 763 mg sodium

Roasted Chickpeas

Can you enjoy a high-protein snack without meat or cheese? With the South Beach Diet you can.

400 g (14 oz) tinned chickpeas, rinsed and drained

Preheat the oven to 180°C/350°F/gas 4.

Spread the chickpeas on an ungreased baking sheet in a single layer. Bake for 50 minutes, or until browned and crisp enough to rattle.

Makes 4 servings

NUTRITION AT A GLANCE
Per serving: Energy 115 cals/485 kJ; 3 g fat (of which 0.5 g saturates), 7 g protein, 16 g carbohydrate (of which 0.5 g sugars), 4 g fibre, 220 mg sodium

CHEF ANDREW ROTHSCHILD

THE FORGE HAS BEEN A LANDMARK MIAMI RESTAURANT FOR DECADES, BUT THIS MUSHROOM 'SOUP' IS ANYTHING BUT OUTDATED!

Wild Mushroom Cappuccino

PHASE 1

1	onion, finely chopped
2	cloves garlic, crushed
2	tablespoons rapeseed (canola) oil
145 g (5 oz)	assorted mushrooms (shiitake, ceps, small portobello or chestnut mushrooms), sliced
1 L (1¾ pints)	chicken stock

30 g (1 oz)	fresh thyme leaves or bunch of thyme stems
1	bay leaf
	salt
	pepper
240 ml (8 fl oz)	cold skimmed milk
1	teaspoon porcini powder (optional)

Sauté the onion and garlic in the oil until translucent. Add the mushrooms and sauté until they begin to caramelize. Add the stock, thyme and bay leaf. Boil to reduce by half.

Strain through a fine conical sieve into a jug. Season with salt and pepper and pour into coffee cups. Froth the cold milk in a cappuccino machine. Spoon the froth on top and sprinkle with the porcini powder.

Makes 4 servings

NUTRITION AT A GLANCE
Per serving: Energy 147 cals/615 kJ; 10 g fat (of which 1 g saturates), 5 g protein, 9 g carbohydrate (of which 7 g sugars), 1.5 g fibre, 688 mg sodium

Spicy Bean Dip

Need a quick party dip? This one's a hit every time. It's excellent with fresh vegetables or wholemeal pitta bread in Phase 2. It's best hot, but it's good cold as well.

400 g (14 oz)	tinned fat-free refried beans or black beans, drained and rinsed
240 ml (8 fl oz)	ffat-free natural yogurt
400 g (14 oz)	tinned chopped tomatoes
1	jalapeño chilli, chopped (wear rubber gloves when handling)
½	teaspoon salt
1	teaspoon ground black pepper
115 g (4 oz)	reduced-fat Cheddar cheese, grated (optional)

Preheat the oven to 160°C/325°F/gas 3.

If using black beans, put them in a large bowl and crush with a fork.

Combine the beans with the yogurt, tomatoes (with juice), chilli, salt and black pepper. Spoon into a 1-litre (2-pint) shallow baking dish. Top with the cheese, if using.

Bake for 10 minutes, or until heated through.

Makes 700 ml (25 fl oz)

NUTRITION AT A GLANCE

Per 2 tablespoons: Energy 90 cals/376 kJ; 3 g fat (of which 1.5 g saturates), 7 g protein, 8 g carbohydrate (of which 3 g sugars), 3 g fibre, 200 mg sodium

Tomato Salsa with Avocado and Onion

Easy to prepare, a salsa like this makes a refreshing dip or a sassy addition to plain chicken, fish or vegetables. Serve with toasted wholemeal pitta triangles (see note) for a Phase 2 snack.

2 tomatoes, finely chopped

½ red onion, chopped

½ avocado, cubed

1 green chilli, seeded and chopped (wear rubber gloves when handling)

2 tablespoons chopped fresh parsley

1 tablespoon red wine vinegar

2 teaspoons grated lime zest

1 teaspoon lime juice

¼ teaspoon ground cumin

assorted prepared fresh vegetables, such as celery sticks, cauliflower florets, cucumber slices

In a large serving bowl, combine the tomatoes, onion, avocado, chilli, parsley, vinegar, lime zest and juice and cumin. Leave to stand for 15 minutes before serving. Serve with the prepared vegetables and pitta triangles for dipping.

Note: to make the pitta triangles, cut wholewheat pitta into triangles and bake at 180°C/350°F/gas 4 until lightly browned.

Makes 6 servings

NUTRITION AT A GLANCE
Per serving: Energy 41 cals/171 kJ; 3 g fat (of which 1 g saturates), 1 g protein, 2 g carbohydrate (of which 1.5 g sugars), 1 g fibre, 4 mg sodium

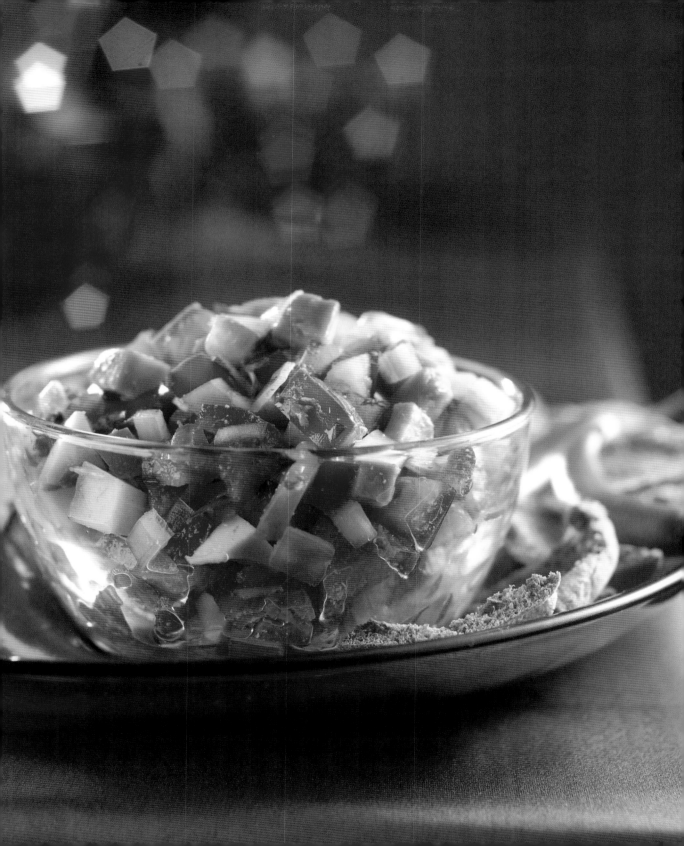

Yogurt Cheese Cucumber Dip

It is easy to make a satiny fresh cheese from yogurt. It is delicious plain or mixed with chopped chives or garlic and stuffed into mushroom caps or cherry tomatoes. Here it's combined with a refreshing cucumber mixture to make a satisfying dip you can scoop up with fresh vegetables.

455 g (1 lb)	fat-free natural yogurt
1	cucumber, grated
120 ml (4 fl oz)	fresh lemon juice
2	cloves garlic, finely chopped
1	tablespoon chopped fresh dill

Line a strainer or sieve with a double layer of cheesecloth and place it over a bowl. Spoon in the yogurt and tie the corners of the cheesecloth together. Let it drain in the refrigerator overnight. Do not allow the strainer to touch the liquid.

Squeeze the yogurt gently and remove it from the cheesecloth. Discard the liquid. Use the yogurt cheese immediately or cover and refrigerate for up to 5 days.

Squeeze the cucumber in a clean tea towel to remove the moisture.

In a large bowl, combine the cucumber, yogurt cheese, lemon juice and garlic. Sprinkle with the dill.

Makes 230 g (8 oz)

NUTRITION AT A GLANCE
Per 2 tablespoons: Energy 45 cals/188 kJ; 0.5 g fat (of which 0 g saturates), 4 g protein, 7 g carbohydrate (of which 6 g sugars), 1 g fibre, 60 mg sodium

MY SOUTH BEACH DIET

'THIS NEW WAY OF EATING HAS LITERALLY SAVED MY LIFE.
The South Beach Diet has saved my life. At 38 years old and 180 kg (more than 28 st), I was desperate to make a change and seriously considering gastric bypass surgery – until I learned about the South Beach Diet.

What really triggered me to lose weight was my partner of 17 years, Dennis. I knew that if I didn't do something about my weight, we wouldn't have many more years to spend with each other.

I started Phase 1 on 23 June. At that time, my cholesterol and blood pressure were way too high, even with medication. In September, I went back to my doctor for a check-up. My weight had dropped to 157 kg (just under 25 st). My cholesterol and blood pressure were well within healthy limits. All my doctor could say was 'Phenomenal . . . phenomenal . . . phenomenal. . . . '

Luckily, I found this new way of life pretty easy from the start. I stayed on Phase 1 for three weeks and lost more than 14 kg (over 2 st), just by following the food suggestions presented in the book. The dramatic weight loss in such a short period of time motivated me to keep going.

I felt good about South Beach because I was learning the right way to fuel my body. I learned how important it is to eat three meals a day with snacks in-between and that the way to lose weight was not skipping meals. It was strange eating a snack when I wasn't very hungry, but I soon realized the importance of it. It kept me from getting famished and overeating later in the day.

In Phase 2, I added wholegrain bread, wholewheat pitta bread, wholewheat pasta, berries and, yes, chocolate back into my diet. I've continued to lose weight at the rate of ½ to 1 kg (1 to 2 lb) a week. Recently, I started walking and now walk 1½ kilometres (1 mile), three times each day. I lost 1.8 kg (4 lb) last week, and my total weight loss after being on the South Beach Diet for only three months is now 25 kg (4 st)!

This new way of eating has literally saved my life. I really believe I'm learning a sensible way to eat that I can live with for ever. My partner is also extremely proud of what I have accomplished so far. I now know we'll have many more years to share together.

Not only do I know I will reach my goal weight, but I also know I'll keep it off this time. – *EDWARD O.*

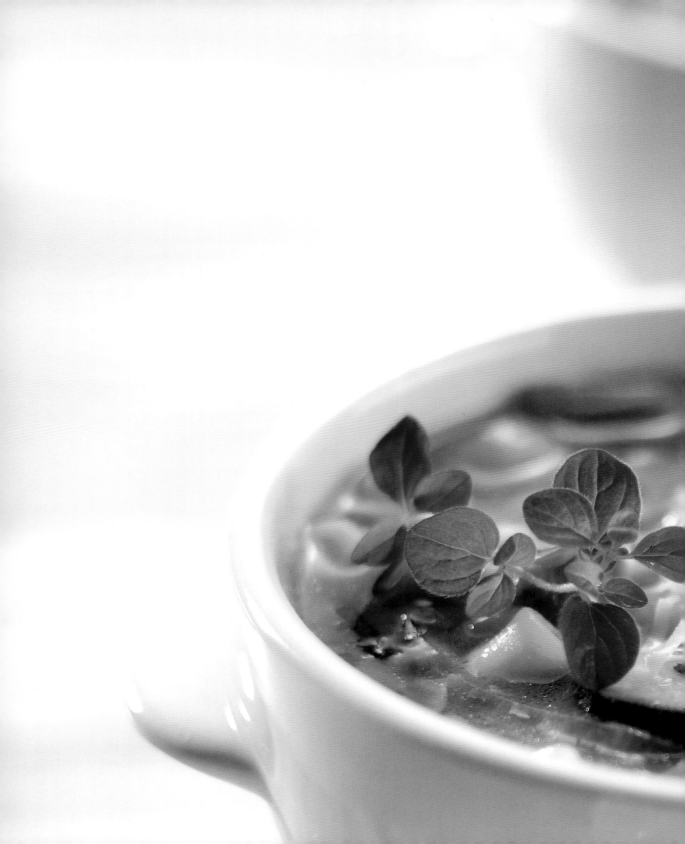

SOUPS

HERE'S WHY HEALTHY SOUPS ARE A GOOD IDEA FOR DIETERS: THE BRAIN DOESN'T EVEN BEGIN GETTING THE MESSAGE THAT YOU'RE FILLING YOUR STOMACH UNTIL 20 MINUTES OR SO AFTER YOU'VE BEGUN TO EAT. SO ANY LOW-CARB FIRST COURSE IS GOOD BECAUSE IT STARTS SENDING THE MESSAGE EARLY. WHEN SERVED AS A STARTER, SOUP EXTENDS THE OVERALL MEAL TIME AND AUTOMATICALLY KEEPS YOU FROM STUFFING YOURSELF LATER IN THE MEAL.

IN PHASE 1 OF THE DIET, I RECOMMEND EITHER CLEAR CHICKEN OR BEEF BROTH OR CONSOMMÉ, GAZPACHO, OR SOUPS WITH LOTS OF VEGETABLES. AFTER THOSE FIRST 2 WEEKS, NEARLY ALL SOUPS ARE SOUTH BEACH–LEGAL, EITHER AS A FIRST COURSE OR AS A MAIN COURSE. THERE'S NO END TO THE COMBINATIONS OF MEAT, FISH, VEGETABLES AND WHOLE GRAINS YOU CAN USE. YOU MAY EVEN INCLUDE MODEST AMOUNTS OF WHOLEWHEAT PASTA OR LONG-COOKING RICE. I'VE INCLUDED SEVERAL RECIPES FOR THICK, CREAMY SOUPS MADE WITHOUT CREAM. YOU'LL NEVER MISS IT!

Chinese-Style Gazpacho

Serve this clever combination of ingredients as a light first course with any variety of other dishes. It's also perfect for a light summer lunch outdoors.

6	tomatoes, seeded and finely chopped
500 ml (18 fl oz)	chicken stock
1	teaspoon dry sherry
2	tablespoons chopped fresh coriander
1	tablespoon light soy sauce
4	spring onions, white part only
4	thin slices fresh ginger
¼	teaspoon Chinese chilli sauce
2	limes

Place the tomatoes in a large saucepan over low heat. Add the stock, sherry, coriander, soy sauce, spring onions and ginger. Bring the mixture to a simmer and cook for 20 minutes. Remove from the heat and leave to cool for a few minutes. Purée in a blender or food processor. Chill.

Just before serving, stir in the chilli sauce. Grate the zest from 1 lime and add it to the soup. Squeeze the juice from both limes into the soup. Serve in chilled bowls.

Makes 6 servings

NUTRITION AT A GLANCE

Per serving: Energy 30 cals/125 kJ; 0.5 g fat (of which 0 g saturates), 2 g protein, 4 g carbohydrate (of which 3 g sugars), 1 g fibre, 391 mg sodium

Chilled Tomato Bisque

This tomato bisque is rich, creamy, tasty — and easy to make.

4	medium tomatoes, peeled, seeded and finely chopped
350 ml (12 fl oz)	V8 juice or vegetable cocktail juice
240 ml (8 fl oz)	buttermilk
1	teaspoon dried basil
¼	teaspoon ground black pepper

Place the tomatoes, vegetable juice or vegetable cocktail juice, buttermilk, basil and pepper in a blender or food processor and process until smooth. Refrigerate for at least 1 hour before serving.

Makes 4 servings

NUTRITION AT A GLANCE
Per serving: Energy 60 cals/250 kJ; 0.5 g fat (of which 0 g saturates), 6 g protein, 9 g carbohydrate (of which 9 g sugars), 1.5 g fibre, 228 mg sodium

ALTHOUGH *PICASSO* IS NOT IN MIAMI, CHEF JULIAN SERRANO IS A PART OF THE ANNUAL SOUTH BEACH WINE AND FOOD FESTIVAL — ONE OF MY FAVOURITE LOCAL EVENTS.

Classic Gazpacho with Avocado Crab Farci

PHASE 3

Gazpacho

685 g (1½ lb)	ripe tomatoes, chopped (reserve ½ tomato for stuffing)
½	large green pepper (capsicum), chopped
½	onion, chopped
½	cucumber, seeded and chopped
2	cloves garlic
480 ml (16 fl oz)	tomato juice
1	tablespoon cumin seeds
4	tablespoons sherry vinegar
4	slices day-old bread
480 ml (16 fl oz)	water
2	tablespoons extra virgin olive oil
	salt and pepper

Stuffed Avocado

2	ripe avocados, rinsed and halved
½	cucumber, seeded and finely chopped
½	onion, finely diced
½	tomato, finely chopped (reserved from gazpacho)
½	green pepper (capsicum), finely chopped
455 g (1 lb)	crabmeat
	cherry tomatoes, to garnish

To make the gazpacho: Put the tomatoes, green pepper, onion, cucumber, garlic, tomato juice, cumin, vinegar, bread, water and oil in a large bowl for 6 hours.

After 6 hours, purée in a blender or food processor and season with salt and pepper to taste. Refrigerate until cold.

To make the stuffed avocados: Remove most of the flesh from each avocado half, leaving a 1 cm (½ in) shell around each.

In a small bowl, mix the avocado flesh, cucumber, onion, tomato and pepper. Divide the mixture among the avocado halves. Top each avocado half with crabmeat.

To serve: Serve in chilled bowls: put a half stuffed avocado in the centre of each bowl and ladle the gazpacho around. Garnish each serving with cherry tomatoes.

Makes 4 servings

NUTRITION AT A GLANCE
Per serving: Energy 509 cals/2130 kJ; 27 g fat (of which 5 g saturates), 32 g protein, 35 g carbohydrate (of which 16 g sugars), 8 g fibre, 1207 mg sodium

Indian Tomato Soup

This fragrant, spicy tomato soup makes an interesting beginning to any meal.

230 g (8 oz)	vine-ripened tomatoes or 400 g (14 oz) tinned chopped tomatoes
2	tablespoons extra virgin olive oil
1	onion, finely chopped
1	green chilli, seeded and finely chopped (wear rubber gloves when handling)
3	cloves garlic, crushed
1	tablespoon tomato purée (concentrate)
1 L (1¾ pints)	vegetable stock
½	teaspoon curry powder
	chopped fresh coriander, to garnish

If using fresh tomatoes, bring a large saucepan of water to the boil over high heat. Cut a small ✕ in the bottom of each tomato and plunge them into the boiling water for 30 seconds each. Remove the tomatoes, place in a bowl of cold water for a few seconds, then drain. When cool enough to handle, peel away the loosened skin. If the skin fails to peel away easily, return the tomatoes to the boiling water for an additional 10 seconds. Remove the cores from the tomatoes and coarsely chop the flesh.

Heat the oil in a large saucepan over medium heat. Add the onion, chilli and garlic and cook for 4 minutes, or until soft. Stir in the fresh or tinned tomatoes and cook, stirring often, for 5 minutes.

In a small bowl, blend the tomato purée with the vegetable broth and add to the saucepan. Add the curry powder and simmer for 7 minutes.

To serve, ladle the hot soup into 4 warmed bowls and garnish with the coriander.

Makes 4 servings

NUTRITION AT A GLANCE
Per serving: Energy 89 cals/372 kJ; 6 g fat (of which 1 g saturates), 3 g protein, 7 g carbohydrate (of which 4 g sugars), 1.5 g fibre, 379 mg sodium

Teriyaki Mushroom Soup with Watercress

Watercress is a member of the mustard family, and it has a slightly bitter flavour that is tempered here with teriyaki sauce, lemon juice and fresh coriander. If you omit the noodles and prepare South Beach Teriyaki Sauce (page 163), you can also enjoy this recipe in Phase 1.

1 L (1¾ pints)	chicken stock
1	tablespoon teriyaki sauce
170 g (6 oz)	mushrooms, thinly sliced
75 g (2½ oz)	watercress, finely chopped
100 g (3½ oz)	bean thread (cellophane) noodles
1	tablespoon lemon juice
1	tablespoon chopped fresh coriander
	pinch of cayenne pepper

Bring the stock and teriyaki sauce to the boil in a 3-litre (5-pint) saucepan over medium-high heat. Reduce the heat to low and stir in the mushrooms, watercress, noodles, lemon juice, coriander and cayenne pepper. Simmer for 7 minutes, or until the noodles and mushrooms are tender. Serve hot.

Makes 6 servings

NUTRITION AT A GLANCE
Per serving: Energy 79 cals/330 kJ; 1.5 g fat (of which 0.5 g saturates), 4 g protein, 12 g carbohydrate (of which 0.5 g sugars), 1 g fibre, 421 mg sodium

Peanut Butter Stew

If you like peanut butter, you'll be nuts about this stew. It's great for lunch or dinner.

2	tablespoons groundnut (peanut) oil
1	large onion, finely chopped
900 g (2 lb)	lean stewing steak, cut into 4 cm (1½ in) pieces
115 g (4 oz)	smooth unsweetened peanut butter
350 ml (12 fl oz)	cold water
5	tablespoons tomato purée (concentrate)
450 ml (15 fl oz)	hot water
1	teaspoon chipotle pepper powder, or ½ teaspoon cayenne pepper and ½ teaspoon liquid smoke or smoked paprika
2	bay leaves
	salt
	freshly ground black pepper

Heat the oil in a heavy saucepan over medium heat. Add the onion and cook for 3 minutes, or until the onion is translucent. Add the steak and cook, stirring occasionally, for 5 minutes, or until the meat is lightly browned on all sides.

In a small bowl, combine the peanut butter with the cold water, then pour it over the meat. Dilute the tomato purée in the hot water and add to the stew. Stir thoroughly. Add the chipotle pepper powder (or cayenne pepper and liquid smoke or smoked paprika), bay leaves and salt and black pepper to taste. Reduce the heat to low, cover and cook, stirring occasionally, for 1 hour, or until the meat is tender. Remove and discard the bay leaves. Serve hot.

Makes 6 servings

NUTRITION AT A GLANCE
Per serving: Energy 336 cals/1406 kJ; 19 g fat (of which 5 g saturates), 35 g protein, 6 g carbohydrate (of which 5 g sugars), 1.5 g fibre, 382 mg sodium

Walnut Soup

A soup is a soup, but this one has all the ingredients of a meal.

1	large fennel bulb, cut into quarters
2	tablespoons extra virgin olive oil
	sea salt
	freshly ground black pepper
1	leek, white part only, sliced
90 g (3 oz)	cauliflower florets
480 ml (16 fl oz)	chicken stock

2	tablespoons dry sherry
60 g (2 oz)	walnuts, toasted and coarsely chopped
30 g (1 oz)	crumbled Stilton or Roquefort cheese
115 g (4 oz)	fat-free natural yogurt
	finely chopped lemon zest
1	tablespoon chopped fresh chives

Preheat the oven to 200°C/400°F/gas 6.

In a small roasting tin, toss the fennel with 1 tablespoon of the oil and sprinkle with the salt and pepper to taste. Bake for 15 minutes, or until tender and golden brown. When cool enough to handle, slice into 1 cm (½ in) strips.

Meanwhile, heat the remaining 1 tablespoon oil in a heavy saucepan over medium–low heat. Add the leek, stirring until coated with oil. Cover and cook for 5 minutes, or until the leek is translucent. Add the cauliflower and stock and bring to the boil. Reduce the heat to low and simmer for 20 minutes, or until the cauliflower is tender. Transfer the mixture to a blender or food processor, add the fennel and process until smooth. Return to the saucepan. Add the sherry and return to a simmer while stirring in the walnuts. Stir in the yogurt and heat gently.

In a small bowl, combine the cheese and lemon zest. Ladle the soup into 4 warmed bowls, add the cheese and chives and serve immediately.

Makes 4 servings

NUTRITION AT A GLANCE

Per serving: Energy 240 cals/1004 kJ; 19 g fat (of which 3.5 g saturates), 8 g protein, 6 g carbohydrate (of which 5 g sugars), 2 g fibre, 775 mg sodium

TALULA RESTAURANT & BAR

210 23rd Street, Miami Beach, Florida

**CHEFS ANDREA CURTO-RANDAZZO
AND FRANK RANDAZZO**

TALULA IS A WARM AND INVITING SPACE, AND ITS OWNERS SAY IT WAS DESIGNED TO FEEL LIKE THEIR HOME. NOW YOU CAN ENJOY THEIR FOOD IN *YOUR* HOME.

Roasted Yellow Pepper Soup with Broad Beans and Cherry Tomatoes

PHASE 1

Soup

5	yellow peppers (capsicums)
2	tablespoons extra virgin olive oil
1	teaspoon salt
½	large onion, chopped
3	cloves garlic, sliced
2	teaspoons ancho or other mild chilli powder
1.2 L (2 pints)	vegetable or chicken stock
	ground white pepper

Garnish

115 g (4 oz)	fresh or frozen baby broad beans or tinned broad beans, rinsed and drained
1	tablespoon extra virgin olive oil
9	cherry tomatoes, halved
1	tablespoon chives, finely chopped
	juice of ½ lemon
	pinch of salt
	pinch of pepper

To make the soup: Preheat the oven to 230°C/450°F/gas 8.

Wash the peppers and place in a large bowl. Toss in 1 tablespoon olive oil and 1 teaspoon salt. Place on a baking sheet and roast in the oven until blistered and brown, about 15 minutes. Remove from the oven and leave to cool.

In a large, heavy saucepan, sauté the onion and garlic in 1 tablespoon olive oil over medium heat until tender, about 5 to 7 minutes, stirring frequently.

Peel the peppers and remove all the seeds. Add peppers and chilli powder to the onions and garlic. Sauté over high heat for 1 minute. Add the stock and bring to the boil. Reduce the heat to medium–low and simmer for 25 to 30 minutes, stirring occasionally.

Purée the soup with a hand blender or in a blender or food processor. Strain through a conical sieve and season with salt and white pepper to taste.

To make the garnish: While the soup is simmering, cook the broad beans in boiling salted water until tender, about 3 minutes. Drain and rinse in ice-cold water. Once cool, drain and remove the outer casing from the beans. Set aside.

To serve: Ladle the soup into 6 warmed bowls. In a small sauté pan, over medium heat, sauté the beans in the olive oil for 1 minute. Add the tomatoes, chives, lemon juice and a pinch of salt and pepper. Spoon the mixture into the middle of each bowl.

Makes 6 servings

NUTRITION AT A GLANCE
Per serving: Energy 124 cals/519 kJ; 6 g fat (of which 1 g saturates), 4 g protein, 13 g carbohydrate (of which 10 g sugars), 4 g fibre, 767 mg sodium

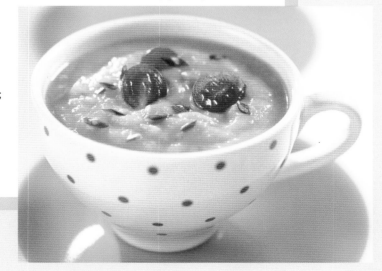

Hearty Minestrone

This recipe calls for ditalini (small tubular pasta), but any other small, shaped pasta will work equally well. If you leave out the pasta, it's a Phase 1 dish.

1 tablespoon extra virgin olive oil	700 ml (1¼ pints) chicken stock
2 leeks, white parts halved lengthwise, rinsed and thinly sliced, green parts chopped	145 g (5 oz) Swiss chard, chopped
	115 g (4 oz) green beans, cut into 2 cm (1 in) pieces
2 sticks of celery, with leaves, thinly sliced	30 g (1 oz) wholewheat ditalini or other small pasta
2 cloves garlic, finely chopped	1 clove garlic, coarsely chopped
¼ teaspoon dried oregano, crushed	4 tablespoons flat-leaved parsley, chopped
¼ teaspoon ground black pepper	60 g (2 oz) courgette (zucchini), sliced
⅛ teaspoon salt	4 teaspoons grated Parmesan cheese
	4 sprigs of oregano, to garnish

Heat the oil in a large saucepan over medium heat. Add the leeks, celery, finely chopped garlic, dried oregano, pepper and salt. Cook, stirring frequently, for 4 minutes, or until the vegetables begin to soften.

Add the stock, Swiss chard, green beans and pasta. Bring to the boil over high heat. Reduce the heat to medium-low, cover and simmer for 8 minutes, or until the vegetables are tender and the pasta is al dente.

Meanwhile, in a cup, combine the coarsely chopped garlic with the parsley. Stir into the soup along with the courgette. Cover and cook for 5 minutes, or until heated through.

Ladle the soup into 4 warmed bowls and top each with 1 teaspoon of the cheese. Garnish with the oregano sprigs.

Makes 4 servings

NUTRITION AT A GLANCE
Per serving: Energy 115 cals/481 kJ; 5 g fat (of which 1.5 g saturates), 6 g protein, 11 g carbohydrate (of which 4 g sugars), 4 g fibre, 262 mg sodium

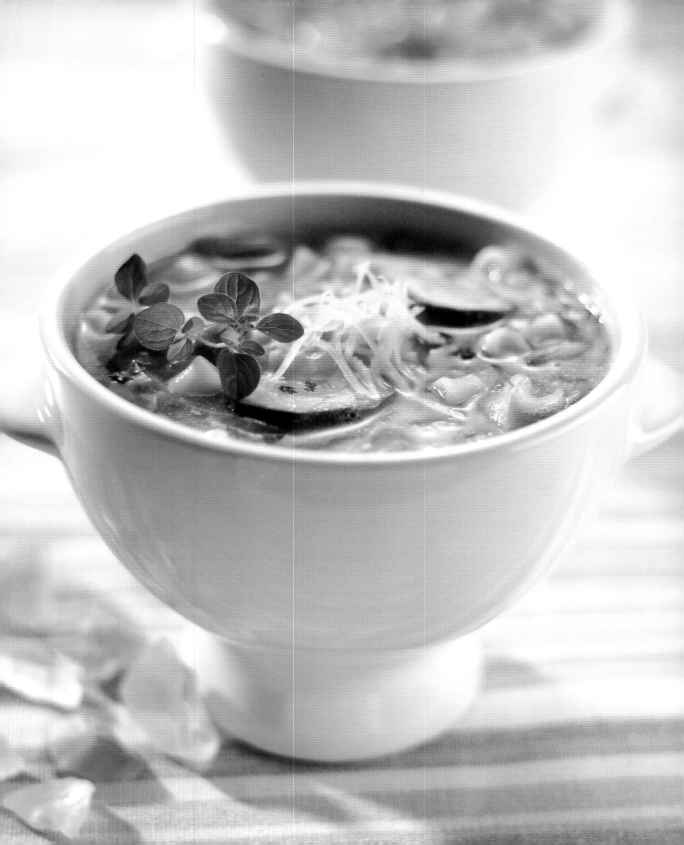

White Bean Soup with Greens

This southern Italian soup features white beans. Use haricot, cannellini, or any other white bean you happen to have.

685g (1½ lb)	Swiss chard, escarole (Batavian endive), or beet greens (spinach beet), trimmed
1.5 L (2½ pints)	chicken stock
1	clove garlic, crushed
200 g (7 oz)	cooked white beans
½	teaspoon salt
⅛	teaspoon ground white pepper
	grated Parmesan cheese, to garnish
	dried chilli flakes, to garnish

Bring a large saucepan of water to the boil over medium–high heat. Add the greens and cook for 7 minutes, or until barely tender. Drain the greens, squeezing out as much water as possible. (This can be done several hours before cooking in the soup. It is not necessary to chop the greens, because they will break apart while they cook in the soup.)

Bring the stock to a simmer in a large saucepan over medium–high heat. Add the garlic and greens. If using canned beans, place them in a strainer and rinse them under cold running water to remove excess sodium. Add the beans to the stock. Simmer gently, partially covered, for 10 minutes. Season with the salt and pepper. (Do not add the salt before the soup has finished cooking, or it may become too salty.)

Ladle into 6 warmed bowls. Pass the cheese and chilli flakes at the table.

Makes 6 servings

NUTRITION AT A GLANCE
Per serving: Energy 103 cals/431 kJ; 4 g fat (of which 1.5 g saturates), 9 g protein, 8 g carbohydrate (of which 2 g sugars), 4 g fibre, 740 mg sodium

Black and White Bean Soup

This soup is truly a meal in itself, with generous servings of both protein and fibre. Enjoy this soup with a crisp salad and a fresh pear for dessert.

145 g (5 oz)	dried black beans
145 g (5 oz)	dried white beans
2	tablespoons extra virgin olive oil
1	onion, chopped
1	small mild fresh chilli, seeded and finely chopped (wear rubber gloves when handling)
1	small stick of celery, chopped
4	cloves garlic, sliced
1½	teaspoons chopped fresh thyme leaves
2 L (3½ pints)	chicken stock
1	teaspoon chilli powder
1	teaspoon ground cumin
1	teaspoon chopped fresh sage
	Roasted Pepper Cream (see page 154)
	fresh coriander leaves, to garnish

Place the black beans and white beans in two separate large bowls, cover with cold water and soak overnight in the refrigerator.

Heat the oil in a large saucepan over medium heat. Add the onion, chilli, celery, garlic and thyme and cook for 8 minutes, or until the vegetables are tender. Transfer half of the vegetables to another large saucepan.

Drain the beans. To the first saucepan, add the black beans, 1 litre (1¾ pints) of stock, the chilli powder and cumin. To the second saucepan, add the white beans, the remaining 1 litre (1¾ pints) stock and the sage. Bring both pans to the boil and cover. Reduce the heat to low. Simmer the black beans for 1½ hours and the white beans for 1 hour or until the beans are tender. Keep both warm over low heat.

To serve, ladle 240 ml (8 fl oz) black bean soup into each of 4 warmed bowls. Tilt the bowls and ladle 240 ml (8 fl oz) white bean soup into the other side of each bowl. Drizzle with the Roasted Pepper Cream and garnish with the coriander leaves.

Makes 4 servings

NUTRITION AT A GLANCE
Per serving: Energy 307 cals/1285 kJ; 8 g fat (of which 1 g saturates), 18 g protein, 42 g carbohydrate (of which 4 g sugars), 8 g fibre, 386 mg sodium

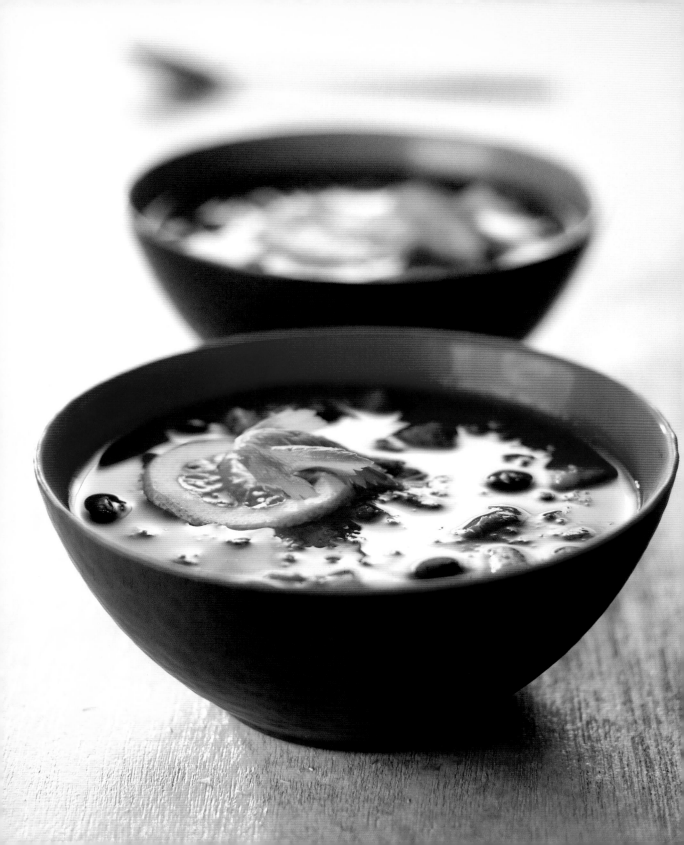

Black Bean Soup

If you like, you can sprinkle a little bit of grated reduced-fat Cheddar cheese over the soup just before serving.

285 g (10 oz)	dried black beans
2	tablespoons extra virgin olive oil
1	onion, chopped
3	cloves garlic, finely chopped
1	stick of celery, with leaves, chopped
1	teaspoon celery seeds
	freshly ground black pepper
	juice of 1½ lemons
1	lemon, sliced paper thin, to garnish
	celery leaves, to garnish

Place the beans in a large bowl, cover with cold water and soak overnight in the refrigerator. The next day, drain the beans and cover with 1.5 litres (2½ pints) of fresh water.

Heat the oil in a large heavy-bottomed saucepan over medium heat. Add the onion, garlic and celery and cook, stirring occasionally, for 5 minutes, or until tender. Add the beans and water and bring to the boil. Reduce the heat to low, cover and simmer for 2 hours, or until the beans are tender.

Transfer half of the beans to a blender or food processor, adding some of the cooking liquid, and process until smooth. Add the celery seeds and black pepper to taste. Return the puréed beans to the pan and heat, stirring, until the soup thickens. Stir in the lemon juice.

Ladle into 6 warmed bowls and garnish with the sliced lemon and celery leaves.

Makes 6 servings

NUTRITION AT A GLANCE
Per serving: Energy 195 cals/816 kJ; 5 g fat (of which 1 g saturates), 12 g protein, 29 g carbohydrate (of which 3 g sugars), 4.5 g fibre, 12 mg sodium

Creole Gumbo

Creole cooking makes ample use of celery, onions, peppers and tomatoes.

2	tablespoons extra virgin olive oil
2	sticks of celery, chopped
½	small onion, chopped
½	green pepper (capsicum), chopped
2	cloves garlic, finely chopped
1½	tablespoons wholemeal flour
2	teaspoons salt
170 g (6 oz)	tinned tomatoes
180 ml (6 fl oz)	South Beach Tomato Sauce (see page 156)
1	tablespoon Worcestershire sauce
115 g (4 oz)	frozen okra, partially thawed and cut into 1 cm (½ in) pieces
145 g (5 oz)	prawns, chopped if large
145 g (5 oz)	crabmeat, flaked
60 ml (2 fl oz)	hot water
1	tablespoon finely chopped fresh parsley

Heat the oil in a 5-litre (8-pint) saucepan over medium–high heat. Add the celery, onion, pepper and garlic and cook, stirring occasionally, for 10 minutes, or until softened. Stir in the flour and salt and cook until the mixture bubbles. Add the tomatoes, South Beach Tomato Sauce and Worcestershire sauce. Reduce the heat to low, cover and simmer for 20 minutes.

Add the okra, prawns, crabmeat, water and parsley and simmer for a further 20 minutes. Serve hot.

Makes 4 servings

NUTRITION AT A GLANCE
Per serving: Energy 209 cals/875 kJ; 8 g fat (of which 1 g saturates), 20 g protein, 14 g carbohydrate (of which 7 g sugars), 3 g fibre, 2145 mg sodium

Buttermilk Salmon Chowder

Yogurt and buttermilk add creaminess to this chunky chowder. Dill, bay leaf and tarragon give subtle flavour accents.

2	turnips, peeled and cut into small cubes
1	onion, chopped
1	stick of celery, chopped
1	teaspoon dill seed
1	bay leaf
500 ml (18 fl oz)	vegetable stock or water
340 g (12 oz)	tinned pink salmon, drained
240 ml (8 fl oz)	buttermilk
230 g (8 oz)	fat-free natural yogurt
1	tablespoon trans-fat-free butter substitute
2	teaspoons Tabasco
¼	teaspoon salt
½	teaspoon ground black pepper
¼	teaspoon dried tarragon

In a large saucepan, combine the turnips, onion, celery, dill seed, bay leaf and stock or water. Bring to the boil over high heat. Reduce the heat to medium and simmer for 12 minutes, or until the vegetables are tender.

Reduce the heat to low. Stir in the salmon, buttermilk, yogurt, butter substitute, Tabasco, salt, black pepper and tarragon. Cook for 5 minutes, or just until heated through. Remove and discard the bay leaf before serving.

Makes 4 servings

NUTRITION AT A GLANCE
Per serving: Energy 255 cals/1067 kJ; 11 g fat (of which 4 g saturates), 26 g protein, 14 g carbohydrate (of which 13 g sugars), 2 g fibre, 926 mg sodium

JOE'S STONE CRAB

11 Washington Avenue, Miami Beach, Florida

CHEF ANDRE BIENVENU

If you're planning a trip to Miami, make sure you go during stone crab season (15 October – 15 May) so you can eat at *Joe's*.

Manhattan Clam Chowder

PHASE 3

30 g (1 oz)	pancetta, chopped
90 g (3 oz)	potatoes, chopped
60 g (2 oz)	yellow onion, chopped
75 g (2½ oz)	carrot, chopped
60 g (2 oz)	celery, chopped
4–5	cloves garlic, chopped
170 g (6 oz)	clams, chopped if large
120 ml (4 fl oz)	bottled or tinned clam juice, or clam and tomato juice
285 g (10 oz)	tinned chopped tomatoes

2	teaspoons tomato purée (concentrate)
2	teaspoons tomato ketchup
1	teaspoon Maggi seasoning
½	teaspoon dried thyme
2	tablespoons plain flour
2	tablespoons cold water
2	tablespoons chopped green pepper (capsicum)
	salt
	black pepper

In a heavy saucepan, cook the pancetta until golden brown. Add the potatoes and cook until lightly browned.

Add the onion, carrot, celery, garlic, clams, clam juice, tomatoes, tomato purée, ketchup, Maggi seasoning and thyme. Simmer for 20 minutes.

In a cup, mix the flour and water to make a paste. Add to the soup and simmer for a further 5 minutes. Add the green pepper and cook for a few more minutes. Add salt and black pepper to taste; serve hot.

Makes 2 servings

NUTRITION AT A GLANCE
Per serving: Energy 274 cals/1147 kJ; 4 g fat (of which 1 g saturates), 25 g protein, 38 g carbohydrate (of which 13 g sugars), 4 g fibre, 1541 mg sodium

Lobster Bisque

Silky and full-flavoured, a bisque makes any meal a celebration.

1	cooked lobster (685–900 g/1½–2 lb)
2	tablespoons rapeseed (canola) oil
1	onion, finely chopped
2	tablespoons wholemeal flour
850 ml (1½ pints)	fish stock
120 ml (4 fl oz)	tomato passata (sieved tomatoes)
60 ml (2 fl oz)	dry sherry
¼	teaspoon salt
300 ml (10 fl oz)	skimmed milk
¼	teaspoon Tabasco
1	teaspoon paprika
1	plum tomato, chopped
2	tablespoons chopped fresh parsley

Remove the lobster flesh and cut into 2.5 cm (1 in) pieces. Using a heavy cleaver, roughly chop the shell and set aside.

Heat the oil in a large saucepan over medium-high heat. Add the onion and the chopped lobster shell and cook, stirring occasionally, for 5 minutes, or until the onion is tender. Stir in the flour and cook, stirring constantly, for 3 minutes, or until lightly browned.

Stir in the stock, passata, sherry and salt and bring to the boil. Reduce the heat to low, cover and simmer for 10 to 15 minutes. Pour through a strainer into a clean saucepan.

Stir in the lobster flesh, milk, Tabasco and paprika. Cook over medium heat for 3 minutes, or until heated through. Stir in the plum tomato and parsley and serve hot.

Makes 4 servings

NUTRITION AT A GLANCE
Per serving: Energy 350 cals/1465 kJ; 12 g fat (of which 2 g saturates), 40 g protein, 17 g carbohydrate (of which 9 g sugars), 2 g fibre, 1213 mg sodium

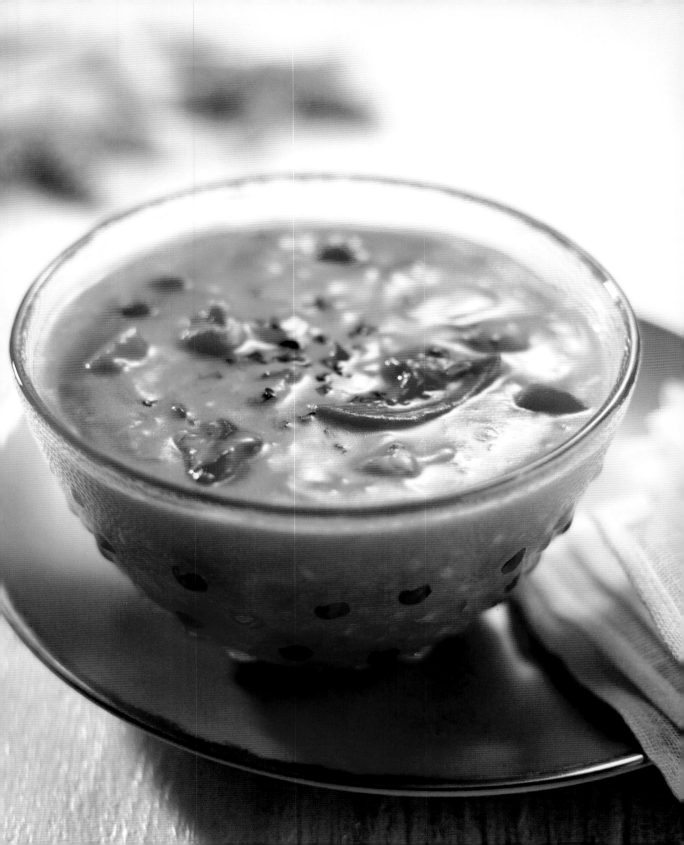

Chicken and Red Lentil Soup

For an extra touch of Indian style, use some shredded unsweetened coconut as an additional garnish.

1	tablespoon extra virgin olive oil
2	small carrots, finely chopped
2	large sticks of celery, finely chopped
½	large onion, sliced
1½	cloves garlic, finely chopped
1	teaspoon curry powder
¼	teaspoon ground ginger
¼	teaspoon ground cumin
¼	teaspoon dried chilli flakes
145 g (5 oz)	red lentils
900 g (2 lb)	boneless, skinless chicken breasts
700 ml (1¼ pints)	chicken stock
1½	teaspoons tomato purée (concentrate)
480 ml (16 fl oz)	water
	sliced spring onion, to garnish

Heat the oil in a large saucepan over medium heat. Add the carrots, celery, onion, garlic, curry powder, ginger, cumin and chilli. Cover and cook for 15 minutes, stirring occasionally, until the vegetables have softened. Stir in the lentils and place the chicken on top. Add the stock.

In a cup, combine the tomato purée with a small amount of the water, then stir into the vegetable mixture. Add the remaining water. Partially cover and simmer for 30 minutes, or until the vegetables are soft and the chicken is cooked through.

Remove the saucepan from the heat. Remove the chicken from the pan and cut into shreds.

Transfer about 450 ml (15 fl oz) of the vegetables and liquid to a blender or food processor and purée until smooth, then return it to the saucepan, along with the shredded chicken.

Divide the soup among 4 warmed bowls and garnish with the spring onion.

Makes 4 servings

NUTRITION AT A GLANCE
Per serving: Energy 437 cals/1829 kJ; 11 g fat (of which 3 g saturates), 60 g protein, 27 g carbohydrate (of which 6 g sugars), 3 g fibre, 551 mg sodium

Chicken and Vegetable Chowder

Move over, chicken noodle soup! A purée of vegetables thickens this sensational chowder. Serve with wholegrain bread to make a hearty one-dish meal.

700 ml (1¼ pints) chicken stock

2 carrots, chopped

2 sticks of celery, chopped

1 onion, chopped

60 g (2 oz) mushrooms, sliced

1 clove garlic, finely chopped

1 teaspoon chopped fresh thyme leaves

¼ teaspoon salt

455 g (1 lb) boneless, skinless chicken breast, cut into 2 cm (¾ in) strips

2 tablespoons trans-fat-free butter substitute

3 tablespoons wholemeal flour

240 ml (8 fl oz) skimmed milk

3 spears asparagus, cut into 2.5 cm (1 in) pieces, or 75 g (2½ oz) broccoli florets

1 tablespoon chopped fresh parsley

¼ teaspoon ground black pepper

In a large saucepan, combine the stock, carrots, celery, onion, mushrooms, garlic, thyme and salt. Bring to the boil over high heat. Reduce the heat to low, cover and simmer for 20 minutes, or until the vegetables are tender. Using a slotted spoon, transfer half of the vegetable mixture to a food processor and process until smooth. Return to the saucepan.

Stir in the chicken, cover and simmer for 15 minutes, or until the chicken is no longer pink.

Melt the butter substitute in a small saucepan over medium heat. Stir in the flour until smooth and cook for 1 minute. Gradually add the milk and cook, stirring constantly, for 3 minutes, or until thickened. Stir into the chicken mixture. Add the asparagus or broccoli, parsley and pepper and cook for 5 minutes, or until heated through. Serve hot.

Makes 4 servings

NUTRITION AT A GLANCE

Per serving: Energy 298 cals/1247 kJ; 10 g fat (of which 5 g saturates), 31 g protein, 21 g carbohydrate (of which 10 g sugars), 3.5 g fibre, 379 mg sodium

MY SOUTH BEACH DIET

I LOVE THE SIMPLICITY OF THIS PLAN.

I've become a walking advertisement for the South Beach Diet. I have lost 16 kg (2½ st) in three months, and everyone who sees me wants to know how I've done it.

Three months ago, I weighed 86 kg (13½ st). At 43 years of age, with a family history of heart disease and diabetes, I was afraid that I wouldn't be around to watch my two precious girls grow up. I weighed 50 kg (less than 8 st) when I was first married, but years of struggling with infertility and two hard-won pregnancies took their toll.

In desperation, I started the Atkins diet even though I had misgivings about all the fat in that plan. Two days later, my mother called me from a health spa where, she said, the South Beach Diet was all the rage. I walked to the bookshop to buy the book and read it that night. The next day, I switched to the South Beach Diet, and I honestly feel like it is a change for life. Of the many things I love about it, foremost is its flexibility. I stuck pretty closely to Phase 1 for the first two weeks and lost 4.5 kg (10 lb)!

Since then, I have successfully gone on holiday, celebrated a birthday with a wonderful dinner that included dessert, and sampled some delicious cakes and pastries from a top French pastry chef. Whenever I do treat myself or stray a bit, I always go back to a South Beach breakfast the next day, and I'm right back on track.

I think one of my greatest reasons for success with this plan is its simplicity. With two small children, it is important to me that there are no points to count, lists of foods to memorize, or special exercises that need to be done.

Right now my exercise is limited to pushing my 1½-year-old daughter in a buggy (stroller) or walking my older daughter to her gymnastics or ice skating classes, and I am still losing weight!

Also, as promised in the diet, I have not had any cravings since my second day on the diet, and I've never been hungry. I really do see this as the way that I will eat, and teach my family to eat, for the rest of my life. – *ELLEN S.*

Vegetable Beef Soup

Some soups are hearty; this soup is good for your heart because of all the fibre from the cabbage, spinach and celery.

2	tablespoons extra virgin olive oil
455 g (1 lb)	stewing beef, trimmed of fat and cut into 3 cm (1¼ in) cubes
1	stick of celery, finely chopped
½	large onion, finely chopped
115 g (4 oz)	green beans, cut into 2–3 cm (1 in) pieces
1.2 L (2 pints)	water
¼	small cabbage, coarsely shredded
90 g (3 oz)	spinach, coarsely shredded
400 g (14 oz)	tinned chopped tomatoes
½	teaspoon salt
	freshly ground black pepper

Heat 2 tablespoons of the oil in a large saucepan over medium–high heat. Add the beef and cook, stirring occasionally, for 8 minutes, or until well browned on all sides and no longer pink in the centre. Using a slotted spoon, transfer to a large bowl lined with paper towels and pat with paper towels to remove excess fat.

Put the saucepan back on the heat and add the celery, onion and green beans and cook, stirring occasionally, for 10 minutes, or until the vegetables are lightly browned. Add the beef, water, cabbage, spinach, tomatoes (with juice) and pepper to taste. Bring to the boil over high heat, stirring frequently. Reduce the heat to low, cover and simmer, stirring occasionally, for 1½ hours, or until the meat is fork-tender. Serve hot.

Makes 4 servings

NUTRITION AT A GLANCE

Per serving: Energy 236 cals/988 kJ; 11 g fat (of which 3 g saturates), 26 g protein, 8 g carbohydrate (of which 7 g sugars), 3 g fibre, 442 mg sodium

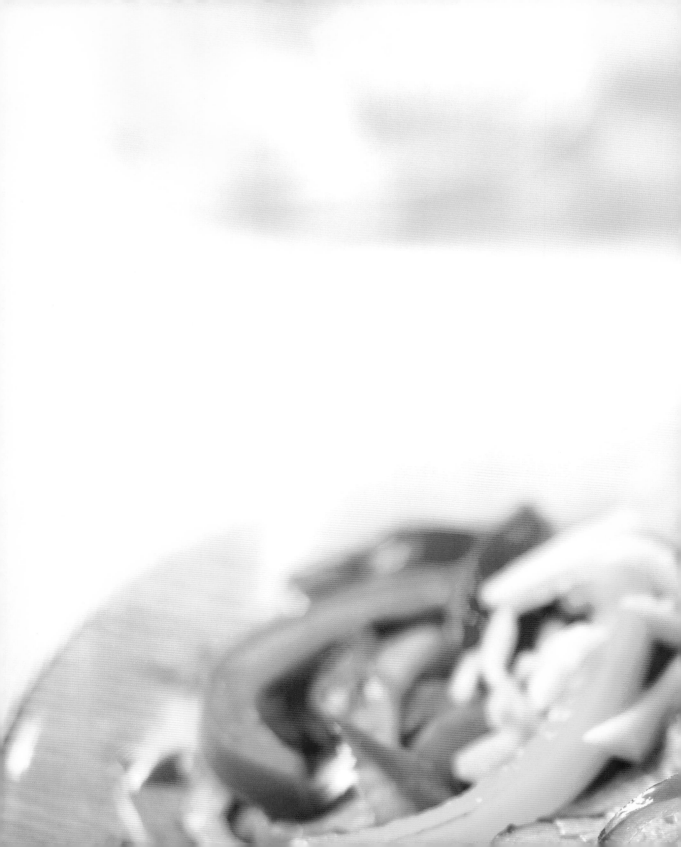

SALADS

For people trying to lose excess weight, there may be nothing more predictable — and less welcome — than suggestions for salads. Our goal was to come up with salads that contain enough protein — meat, fish, or cheese — to truly satisfy your hunger. Vegetarians can add beans instead of meat for bulk, flavour and protein. Salads are also a good way to use leftover meat or fish from the day before. We've also created some unusual side salads to help you expand your idea of the vegetables in a salad beyond lettuce or spinach.

We steer clear of low-fat dressings, which usually contain sugars or starches. Instead, feel free to use a good vinaigrette, or make your own dressing from olive oil and vinegar or lemon juice. Mayonnaise is also fine, since most mayo is made from a healthy oil, eggs, vinegar and seasonings. It's also becoming easier to find commercially made sugar-free dressings.

Tropical Prawn and Black Bean Salad

Colourful tropical fruits enhance this prawn and bean salad. It's terrific for lunch or a light dinner.

Jicama (also known as yam bean) is a juicy, crunchy tuber, usually eaten raw or stir-fried. If you can't find it in the shops, you could substitute sliced water chestnuts.

455 g (1 lb)	medium cooked prawns, peeled and deveined
1	tin (400 g/14 oz) black beans, rinsed and drained
1	ripe papaya, peeled, halved, seeded and chopped
2	kiwi fruit, peeled and sliced
1	jicama, peeled and cut into thin strips
½	medium red onion, thinly sliced
8	tablespoons chopped fresh coriander leaves
4	tablespoons extra virgin olive oil

On 4 serving plates, arrange the prawns, beans, papaya, kiwi fruit, jicama and onion. Sprinkle with the coriander and drizzle with the oil.

Makes 4 servings

NUTRITION AT A GLANCE

Per serving: Energy 365 cals/1528 kJ; 14 g fat (of which 2 g saturates), 34 g protein, 27 g carbohydrate (of which 10 g sugars), 6 g fibre, 1600 mg sodium

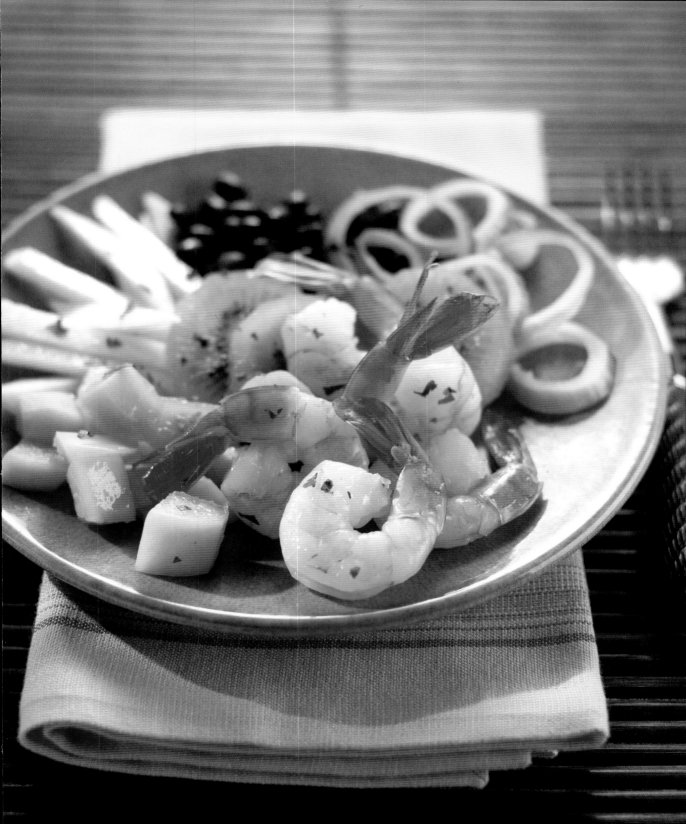

AZUL IS A DRAMATIC DINING SPACE, WITH A WHITE MARBLE–CLAD OPEN KITCHEN AND PICTURESQUE BAY VIEWS FROM ITS FLOOR-TO-CEILING WINDOWS. AND THE FOOD IS AS SPECTACULAR AS THE VIEW.

Shaved Fennel Salad
with Seared Tuna and Parmesan

PHASE 1

Salad

- 1 fennel bulb, shaved paper thin with a mandolin
- 2 tablespoons extra virgin olive oil
- 2 tablespoons fresh lemon juice
- ⅛ teaspoon chopped fresh thyme leaves
- 1 teaspoon chopped fresh flat-leaved parsley
- 20 g (¾ oz) Parmesan cheese, shaved paper thin with a potato peeler

Tuna

- ¼ teaspoon salt
- 1 tablespoon pink peppercorns
- 115 g (4 oz) fresh sushi quality tuna
- 1½ teaspoons extra virgin olive oil

To make the salad: Mix the fennel, oil, lemon juice, thyme, parsley and cheese. Set aside in a cool place.

To sear the tuna: Sprinkle the salt and peppercorns on the tuna. Place a sauté pan over high heat and add the olive oil. Place the tuna in the pan and cook for 30 seconds to 1 minute on each side. Remove from the pan and slice into 5 pieces.

Place the fennel salad on a plate and place the slices of tuna in the centre. Serve immediately.

Makes 1 serving

NUTRITION AT A GLANCE
Per serving: Energy 500 cals/2093 kJ; 40 g fat (of which 10 g saturates), 30 g protein, 3 g carbohydrate (of which 3 g sugars), 4 g fibre, 1124 mg sodium

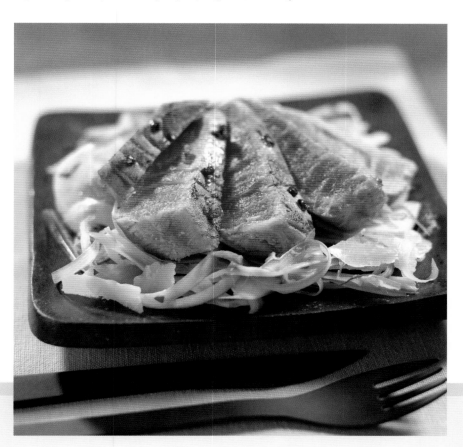

Tuna and Bean Salad

With the saltiness of the capers and the smoothness of the yogurt and mayonnaise, this tuna salad really comes to life. Enjoy it for a satisfying lunch.

2	bunches watercress, tough ends trimmed
60 ml (2 fl oz)	water
1	clove garlic, thinly sliced
340 g (12 oz)	tinned tuna, packed in water, drained and flaked
115 g (4 oz)	tinned cannellini beans, rinsed and drained
¼	white onion, finely chopped
90 g (3 oz)	roasted red pepper (capsicum), chopped
3	tablespoons mayonnaise
2	tablespoons fat-free natural yogurt
1	tablespoon red wine vinegar
1½	teaspoons rinsed and drained capers
	salt
	ground black pepper

Coarsely chop half the watercress stems. Rinse and dry the remaining watercress sprigs and set aside.

In a small saucepan, combine the chopped stems, water and garlic. Bring to the boil over medium-high heat. Reduce the heat to low. Cover and simmer until the watercress stems are bright green, about 1 to 2 minutes. Drain and place in a large bowl. Add the tuna, beans, onion and roasted pepper and toss to mix well.

In a blender or food processor, combine the mayonnaise, yogurt, vinegar, capers, and salt and black pepper to taste. Purée until smooth.

Serve the tuna mixture on the reserved watercress sprigs. Drizzle with the dressing.

Makes 4 servings

NUTRITION AT A GLANCE

Per serving: Energy 295 cals/1235 kJ; 18 g fat (of which 3 g saturates), 25 g protein, 8 g carbohydrate (of which 4 g sugars), 3 g fibre, 752 mg sodium

Chicken Salad with Wonton Crisps

You'll love the sweet-and-sour taste of this crunchy chicken salad. Wonton wrappers and traditional Chinese ingredients provide a taste of the Orient.

8	wonton wrappers, cut into 5 mm (¼ in) strips
4	tablespoons rice vinegar or white wine vinegar
2	tablespoons hoisin sauce
2	tablespoons rapeseed (canola) oil
¼	teaspoon sesame oil
1	tablespoon grated fresh ginger
1	clove garlic, finely chopped
¼	teaspoon dried chilli flakes
400 g (14 oz)	mixed salad leaves
100 g (3½ oz)	bean sprouts
230 g (8 oz)	cooked chicken breast, shredded
1	carrot, grated
2	spring onions, thinly sliced

Preheat the oven to 200°C/400°F/gas 6. Coat a baking sheet with cooking spray.

Separate the wonton strips and place them on the prepared baking sheet. Coat them lightly with cooking spray. Bake for 3 minutes, or until golden brown and crisp. Remove and set aside.

In a large bowl, whisk together the vinegar, hoisin sauce, rapeseed oil, sesame oil, ginger, garlic and chilli flakes. Add the salad leaves, bean sprouts, chicken, carrot, spring onions and wonton strips. Toss gently to mix and serve immediately.

Makes 4 servings

NUTRITION AT A GLANCE

Per serving: Energy 240 cals/1004 kJ; 9 g fat (of which 1 g saturates), 20 g protein, 16 g carbohydrate (of which 4 g sugars), 2 g fibre, 500 mg sodium

Smoked Chicken Salad
with Raspberry-Balsamic Vinaigrette

If you need a meal in minutes, this is just what you're looking for.

4	tablespoons sugar-free raspberry jam or no-added-sugar raspberry fruit spread
3	tablespoons extra virgin olive oil
4	tablespoons balsamic vinegar
340 g (12 oz)	boneless smoked chicken breast, cut into 8 cm (3 in) strips
400 g (14 oz)	mixed salad leaves
250 g (9 oz)	fresh raspberries
30 g (1 oz)	sliced almonds, toasted

Put the fruit spread, oil and vinegar in a screw-topped jar, close the lid tightly and shake vigorously.

In a large bowl, gently toss the chicken with the dressing. Line a large platter or bowl with the salad leaves. Top with the chicken mixture, raspberries and almonds. (Or, if desired, place the chicken, raspberries and almonds on the salad leaves and serve the dressing on the side or drizzled over the top.)

Makes 4 servings

NUTRITION AT A GLANCE
Per serving: Energy 326 cals/1364 kJ; 17 g fat (of which 3 g saturates), 29 g protein, 15 g carbohydrate (of which 14 g sugars), 3 g fibre, 700 mg sodium

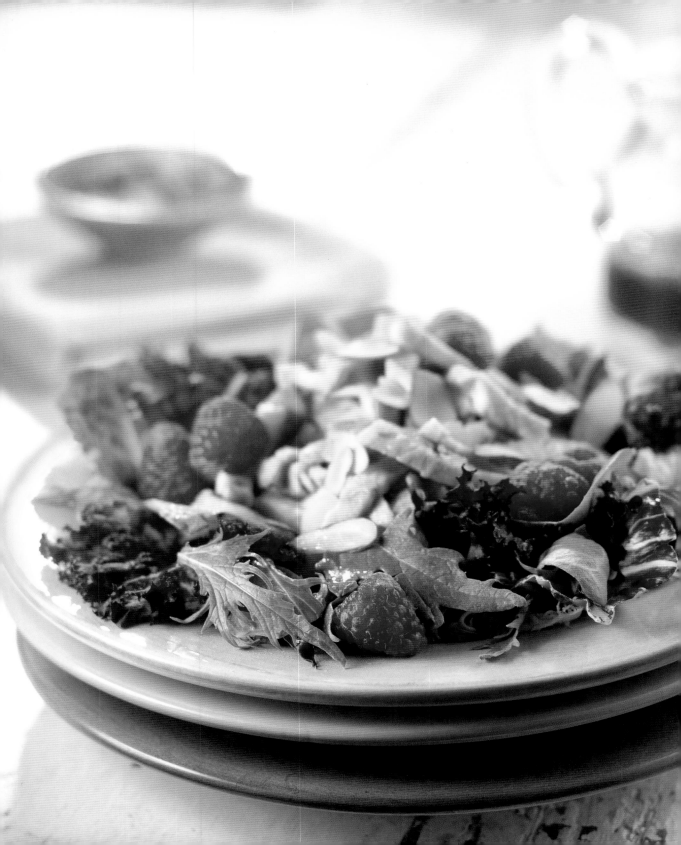

Creamy Chicken Salad

This salad is so simple to make, you'll enjoy preparing it for any occasion.

180 ml (6 fl oz)	fat-free natural yogurt
3	spring onions, finely chopped
1	tablespoon finely chopped fresh parsley
½	teaspoon grated lemon zest
	salt
	ground black pepper
425 g (15 oz)	cooked chicken breast, shredded
8	large lettuce leaves

In a medium bowl, combine the yogurt, spring onions, parsley, lemon zest and salt and pepper to taste. Toss well to blend. Add the chicken and toss to coat. Serve on a bed of lettuce leaves.

Makes 4 servings

NUTRITION AT A GLANCE

Per serving: Energy 203 cals/850 kJ; 5 g fat (of which 2 g saturates), 35 g protein, 4 g carbohydrate (of which 3 g sugars), 0.5 g fibre, 284 mg sodium

Frisée Salad with Blue Cheese and Walnuts

A fruity vinaigrette with a Dijon tang is the perfect complement to the sprinkling of walnuts and blue cheese.

Raspberry Vinaigrette

- 1 tablespoon no-added-sugar raspberry fruit spread
- 8 tablespoons balsamic vinegar
- 1½ teaspoons walnut or rapeseed (canola) oil
- ½ teaspoon Dijon mustard

Salad

- 4 tablespoons red wine
- 1 pear, cored and chopped
- 230 g (8 oz) curly endive (frisée) or mixed salad leaves
- 2 tablespoons toasted walnuts, chopped
- 2 tablespoons crumbled blue cheese
  salt
  ground black pepper

To make the raspberry vinaigrette: Place the fruit spread in a small microwaveable bowl and microwave on high power for 1 minute, or until melted. Whisk in the vinegar, oil and mustard.

To make the salad: Put the wine and pear in a small saucepan over medium-high heat. Cook, stirring often, for 4 minutes, or until the liquid has evaporated.

Divide the frisée or salad leaves among 4 plates. Sprinkle with the walnuts and blue cheese. Sprinkle with salt and pepper to taste. Divide the pear among the plates. Drizzle with the raspberry vinaigrette.

Makes 4 servings

NUTRITION AT A GLANCE

Per serving: Energy 150 cals/628 kJ; 10 g fat (of which 2 g saturates), 3 g protein, 7 g carbohydrate (of which 7 g sugars), 1 g fibre, 151 mg sodium

Chinese Beef and Pepper Salad

Leftover roast beef gets a cool new look.

80 ml (3 fl oz)	light soy sauce
2	tablespoons extra virgin olive oil
1	tablespoon dry sherry
2	teaspoons sugar substitute
1	teaspoon ground ginger
1	small clove garlic, finely chopped
455 g (1 lb)	leftover roast beef, trimmed of all visible fat and cut into slivers about 3 mm (⅛ in) wide and 3 cm (1¼ in) long
1	red pepper (capsicum), cut into very thin slivers
2	spring onions, sliced

In a small bowl whisk together the soy sauce, oil, sherry, sugar substitute, ginger and garlic. Add the beef and toss to coat. Cover and refrigerate for at least an hour, or up to 1 day.

Drain the beef and reserve the marinade. Place the beef in a serving bowl and toss with the pepper and spring onions. Serve with the reserved marinade on the side.

Makes 4 servings

NUTRITION AT A GLANCE
Per serving: Energy 302 cals/1264 kJ; 16 g fat (of which 5 g saturates), 34 g protein, 5 g carbohydrate (of which 2 g sugars), 1 g fibre, 1214 mg sodium

Layered Salad with Avocado-Lime Dressing

If you're looking for a cool, refreshing lunch this summer, you've found it. Make this the night before, keep it in the refrigerator, and when you're ready, it's ready.

Avocado-Lime Dressing

80 ml (3 fl oz)	lime juice
4	tablespoons chopped fresh coriander
1	spring onion, finely chopped
1	tablespoon extra virgin olive oil
1	teaspoon sugar substitute
½	teaspoon salt
3	ripe avocados, peeled and pitted
120 ml (4 fl oz)	salsa (not too chunky)
2	tablespoons lemon juice

Salad

145 g (5 oz)	cherry tomatoes, halved
75 g (2½ oz)	mixed salad leaves
1	large yellow pepper (capsicum), chopped
145 g (5 oz)	cauliflower florets
145 g (5 oz)	cooked turkey ham or lean boiled ham, chopped
115 g (4 oz)	cooked or tinned chickpeas
4	tablespoons sliced black olives
	finely chopped yellow pepper (capsicum), to garnish

To make the avocado-lime dressing: In a small bowl, combine the lime juice, coriander, spring onion, oil, sugar substitute and salt. Add the avocados and mash to incorporate. Stir in the salsa and lemon juice.

To make the salad: In a large glass salad bowl, arrange the tomatoes, cut sides down. Place the salad leaves over the tomatoes. Top with the pepper, then the cauliflower, turkey or ham and chickpeas. Spoon over half of the dressing. Top the dish with the olives and garnish with chopped yellow pepper. Serve with the remaining dressing on the side.

Makes 4 servings

NUTRITION AT A GLANCE

Per serving: Energy 373 cals/1561 kJ; 30 g fat (of which 6 g saturates), 14 g protein, 12 g carbohydrate (of which 6 g sugars), 8 g fibre, 1275 mg sodium

Pork and Pepper Salad

If you want to use leftover pork (or chicken) and roasted peppers from a jar instead of starting with fresh, just warm them in the microwave.

1	red pepper (capsicum)
1	green pepper (capsicum)
1	yellow pepper (capsicum)
230 g (8 oz)	lean pork tenderloin
3	tablespoons extra virgin olive oil
1	red onion, thinly sliced
145 g (5 oz)	red or green cabbage, thinly sliced
2	sticks of celery, thinly sliced
¾	teaspoon salt
½	teaspoon ground black pepper
1	tablespoon balsamic vinegar
30 g (1 oz)	reduced-fat Cheddar or mozzarella cheese, grated (optional)

Preheat the grill. Place the peppers on the grill and cook 10 cm (4 in) from the heat, turning occasionally, until the skin is blistered and browned all over. Place in a paper bag, seal, and set aside for 5 minutes, or until cool enough to handle. Remove, halve, and discard the skin, ribs and seeds. Cut the peppers into strips.

Place the pork on the grill pan and cook for 12 minutes, turning once, or until a thermometer inserted into the centre reaches 70°C/155°F and the juices run clear. Leave to stand for 10 minutes before cutting into thin slices.

Warm 1 tablespoon of the oil in a frying pan over medium heat. Add the onion, cabbage, celery, ½ teaspoon of the salt and ⅛ teaspoon of the black pepper. Cook, stirring frequently, for 10 minutes, or until tender.

Meanwhile, whisk together the remaining 2 tablespoons of olive oil with the balsamic vinegar and season with the remaining salt and pepper.

Divide the cabbage mixture among 4 plates. Arrange the peppers and pork on top. Drizzle each with the dressing and sprinkle with cheese, if using.

Makes 4 servings

NUTRITION AT A GLANCE
Per serving: Energy 249 cals/1042 kJ; 14 g fat (of which 3 g saturates), 22 g protein, 9 g carbohydrate (of which 8 g sugars), 3 g fibre, 501 mg sodium

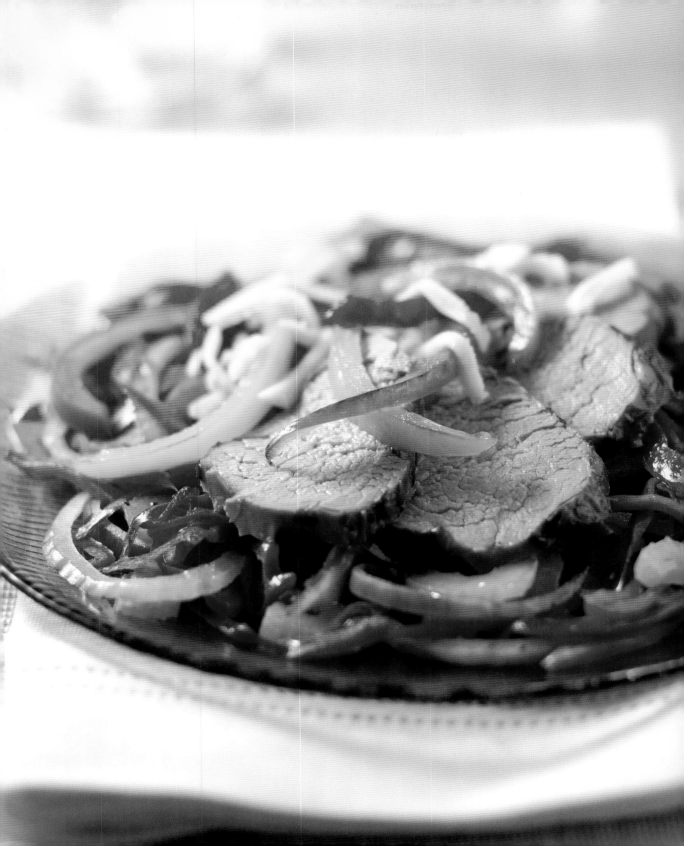

Mixed Salad with Creamy Poppy Seed Dressing

Poppy seed dressing is a delightfully sweet and nutty way to top a salad. To enhance the seeds' flavour, lightly toast them in a small dry frying pan for 2 to 3 minutes before adding them to the dressing.

Dressing

115 g (4 oz)	fat-free natural yogurt
2	tablespoons orange juice
2	teaspoons poppy seeds
½	teaspoon cider vinegar
	pinch of ground black pepper

Salad

1	red-leaved lettuce, coarsely torn
1	bunch watercress
8	cherry tomatoes, halved

To make the dressing: In a small bowl, whisk together the yogurt, orange juice, poppy seeds, vinegar and pepper.

To make the salad: In a salad bowl, combine the lettuce, watercress and tomatoes. Add the dressing and toss gently.

Makes 4 servings

NUTRITION AT A GLANCE

Per serving: Energy 64 cals/268 kJ; 2 g fat (of which 0.5 g saturates), 5 g protein, 7 g carbohydrate (of which 6 g sugars), 2 g fibre, 27 mg sodium

Green Bean and Red Onion Salad

A red onion sauté makes a colourful splash over fresh green beans and cucumber.

455 g (1 lb)	small green beans, steamed and chilled
½	cucumber, seeded and cut into matchsticks
1	red onion, sliced and separated into rings
1–2	cloves garlic, finely chopped
1½	tablespoons extra virgin olive oil
2	tablespoons red wine vinegar
1	tablespoon water
½	teaspoon sugar substitute

In a large bowl, combine the beans and cucumber.

In a small frying pan, sauté the onion and garlic in 1 tablespoon of the oil until tender but not browned. Stir in the vinegar, water and sugar substitute and simmer for 2 minutes, stirring until the sugar substitute is dissolved. Stir in the remaining oil. Spoon the onion dressing over the bean mixture. Serve immediately.

Makes 6 servings

NUTRITION AT A GLANCE
Per serving: Energy 33 cals/138 kJ; 0.5 g fat (of which 0 g saturates), 2 g protein, 6 g carbohydrate (of which 4 g sugars), 2 g fibre, 3 mg sodium

PACIFIC TIME

915 Lincoln Road, Miami Beach, Florida

CHEF JONATHAN EISMANN

PACIFIC TIME IS A WELL-KNOWN PAN-ASIAN RESTAURANT ON MIAMI'S CAR-FREE LINCOLN ROAD. WINDOW SHOPPING AT NEIGHBOURING BOUTIQUES AND GALLERIES IS A FAVOURITE PRE- OR POST-DINNER ACTIVITY.

Chinese Vegetable Salad with Feta

PHASE 1

Dressing

4	tablespoons Chinese black vinegar or white rice vinegar or balsamic vinegar
2	tablespoons strong brewed dark tea
2	tablespoons lime juice
2	tablespoons finely chopped fresh chives
2	tablespoons finely chopped lemongrass

Salad

230 g (8 oz)	Chinese long beans or green beans, cut into 1 cm (½ in) pieces
145 g (5 oz)	feta cheese, crumbled
100 g (3½ oz)	bean sprouts
2	spring onions, green parts only, finely chopped
1	cucumber, peeled, seeded and cut into 5 mm (¼ in) cubes
1	red pepper (capsicum), cut into 5 mm (¼ in) strips
	salt
	ground white pepper

To make the dressing: In a medium bowl, combine the vinegar, tea, lime juice, chives and lemongrass.

To make the salad: Blanch the beans in boiling water for about 2 minutes.

In a large bowl, combine the beans with the cheese, bean sprouts, spring onions, cucumber and pepper. Mix with the dressing. Adjust the seasoning to taste with salt and ground white pepper.

Chill before serving.

Makes 4 servings

NUTRITION AT A GLANCE
Per serving: Energy 143 cals/598 kJ; 8 g fat (of which 5 g saturates), 9 g protein, 9 g carbohydrate (of which 8 g sugars), 3 g fibre, 824 mg sodium

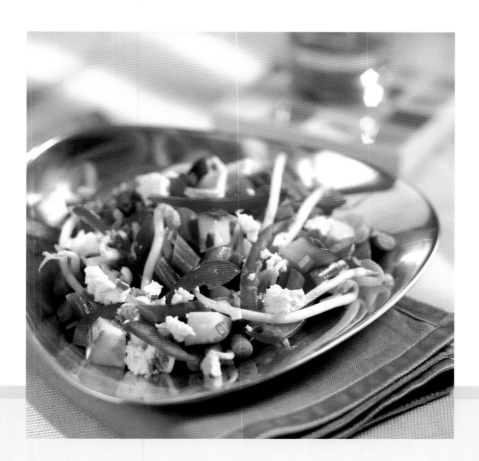

Sesame Mangetout and Asparagus Salad

Mangetouts (snow peas) and sesame are a natural combination. Adding fresh asparagus makes for a very elegant salad. Serve this alongside a main dish, or enjoy it as a light lunch.

285 g (10 oz)	cooked brown rice
2	tablespoons rapeseed (canola) oil
2	teaspoons sesame oil
3	tablespoons light soy sauce
230 g (8 oz)	mangetouts (snow peas), trimmed and cooked
230 g (8 oz)	fresh asparagus, trimmed and cooked
3	tablespoons sesame seeds, toasted
3	spring onions, sliced
¼	teaspoon dried chilli flakes

In a large serving bowl, toss the rice with both oils and the soy sauce. Stir in the mangetouts, asparagus and sesame seeds and toss to combine. Sprinkle with the spring onions and chilli flakes.

Makes 6 servings

NUTRITION AT A GLANCE
Per serving: Energy 164 cals/686 kJ; 8 g fat (of which 1 g saturates), 6 g protein, 18 g carbohydrate (of which 2 g sugars), 2 g fibre, 432 mg sodium

Broad Bean Salad

Broad beans provide the protein in this attractive green salad.

50 g (1¾ oz)	rocket
115 g (4 oz)	mixed salad leaves
400 g (14 oz)	frozen baby broad beans, or tinned broad beans, rinsed and drained
¼	red onion, thinly sliced
	South Beach Green Goddess Dressing (see page 158)

If using frozen beans, cook them in boiling water for 3 minutes. Drain, rinse in cold water, then drain well. In a large bowl, combine the rocket, salad leaves, beans and onion and toss thoroughly. Serve with South Beach Green Goddess dressing.

Makes 4 servings

NUTRITION AT A GLANCE

Per serving: Energy 140 cals/586 kJ; 6 g fat (of which 1 g saturates), 8 g protein, 13 g carbohydrate (of which 3 g sugars), 7 g fibre, 79 mg sodium

Artichoke Salad with Olives

Using tinned or frozen artichoke hearts and a jar of roasted peppers streamlines the preparation time, so you can have the salad ready in a snap.

4	tablespoons mayonnaise
1½	tablespoons extra virgin olive oil
2	teaspoons lemon juice
⅛	teaspoon salt
⅛	teaspoon ground black pepper
285 g (10 oz)	frozen artichoke hearts, thawed and chopped, or artichoke hearts in olive oil, drained and chopped
90 g (3 oz)	roasted red pepper (capsicum), chopped
1	stick of celery, chopped
4	tablespoons chopped fresh basil
8	large black olives, pitted and halved
6	lettuce leaves

In a small bowl, whisk together the mayonnaise, olive oil, lemon juice, salt and black pepper.

In a large serving bowl, combine the artichokes, roasted pepper, celery, basil and olives. Stir in the dressing. Cover and refrigerate until ready to serve.

Put a lettuce leaf on each of 6 plates. Spoon the artichoke mixture onto the lettuce.

Makes 6 servings

NUTRITION AT A GLANCE

Per serving: Energy 185 cals/774 kJ; 19 g fat (of which 3 g saturates), 2 g protein, 3 g carbohydrate (of which 2 g sugars), 1 g fibre, 234 mg sodium

Mixed Vegetable Salad

This salad is full of colour, texture and flavour. It is also delicious topped with cold chicken or prawns.

60 g (2 oz)	fresh green beans cut into lengths
½	carrot, cut into matchsticks
60 g (2 oz)	fresh asparagus, chopped
45 g (1½ oz)	frozen peas
30 g (1 oz)	spinach, torn
½	small fennel bulb, thinly sliced
½	tomato, chopped
45 g (1½ oz)	white mushrooms, sliced
30 g (1 oz)	curly endive (frisée), shredded
½	courgette (zucchini), sliced
¼	cucumber, thinly sliced
30 g (1 oz)	radishes, sliced
8	tablespoons Herb Vinaigrette (see page 159)
1	head of chicory
	chopped fresh coriander, to garnish

Bring a saucepan of water to the boil. Add the green beans and boil for 2 minutes. Add the carrot and cook for 2 minutes. Add the asparagus and peas and cook for a further 2 minutes. Drain well and rinse in cold water. Drain again.

In a large salad bowl, combine the spinach, fennel, tomato, mushrooms, curly endive, courgette, cucumber and radishes. Add the cooked vegetables and the Herb Vinaigrette. Toss well to coat all the vegetables.

To serve, line a platter with the chicory leaves, then spoon the vegetables on top. Sprinkle the coriander over the top to garnish.

Makes 4 servings

NUTRITION AT A GLANCE

Per serving: Energy 142 cals/594 kJ; 11 g fat (of which 2 g saturates), 3 g protein, 7 g carbohydrate (of which 4 g sugars), 3 g fibre, 187 mg sodium

Tomato and Mozzarella Salad

Tomato and fresh basil are a classic combination in Italian cuisine. If you don't have time to roast fresh peppers, you can use roasted peppers in olive oil from a jar; drain and pat them dry with paper towels before using.

1	tablespoon balsamic vinegar
1	teaspoon extra virgin olive oil
1	teaspoon flaxseed oil
1	clove garlic, finely chopped
¼	teaspoon salt
⅛	teaspoon ground black pepper
2	large red peppers (capsicums), halved and seeded
2	large tomatoes, cut into 1 cm (½ in) slices
60 g (2 oz)	mozzarella cheese, cut into 4 slices
4–6	tablespoons fresh basil leaves, cut into thin strips

Preheat the grill. Coat the grill rack with cooking spray.

In a cup, whisk together the vinegar, olive oil, flaxseed oil, garlic, salt and black pepper. Set aside.

Place the peppers, skin side up, on the prepared grill rack. Grill, without turning, for 10 minutes, or until the skins are blackened and blistered in spots.

Place the peppers in a paper bag and seal. Leave for 10 minutes, or until cool enough to handle. Peel the skin from the peppers and discard. Cut the peppers into 1 cm (½ in) strips.

Arrange the tomato slices on a platter. Place the cheese slices over the tomatoes. Scatter the pepper strips on top and sprinkle with the basil. Drizzle the dressing over the salad. Leave for at least 15 minutes to allow the flavours to blend before serving.

Makes 4 servings

NUTRITION AT A GLANCE
Per serving: Energy 91 cals/380 kJ; 5 g fat (of which 2 g saturates), 4 g protein, 7 g carbohydrate (of which 6 g sugars), 2 g fibre, 419 mg sodium

Sweet Potato Salad

Here's a healthy alternative to traditional potato salad. Try it at your next picnic or barbecue.

685 g (1½ lb)	sweet potatoes, scrubbed
1	large apple, peeled, cored and cubed
1	large stick of celery, chopped
1	tablespoon orange juice
1	tablespoon extra virgin olive oil
2	teaspoons cider vinegar
1	teaspoon sugar substitute
	pinch of salt

Place the sweet potatoes in a large saucepan and cover with water. Bring to the boil over medium heat and cook for 20 to 30 minutes, or until tender. Drain and cool. Peel and cut into cubes.

In a large bowl, combine the sweet potatoes, apple and celery.

In a small bowl, whisk together the orange juice, oil, vinegar, sugar substitute and salt. Pour the mixture over the potato mixture and toss to coat. Cover and refrigerate until ready to serve.

Makes 4 servings

NUTRITION AT A GLANCE
Per serving: Energy 194 cals/812 kJ; 4 g fat (of which 0.5 g saturates), 2 g protein, 41 g carbohydrate (of which 15 g sugars), 5 g fibre, 269 mg sodium

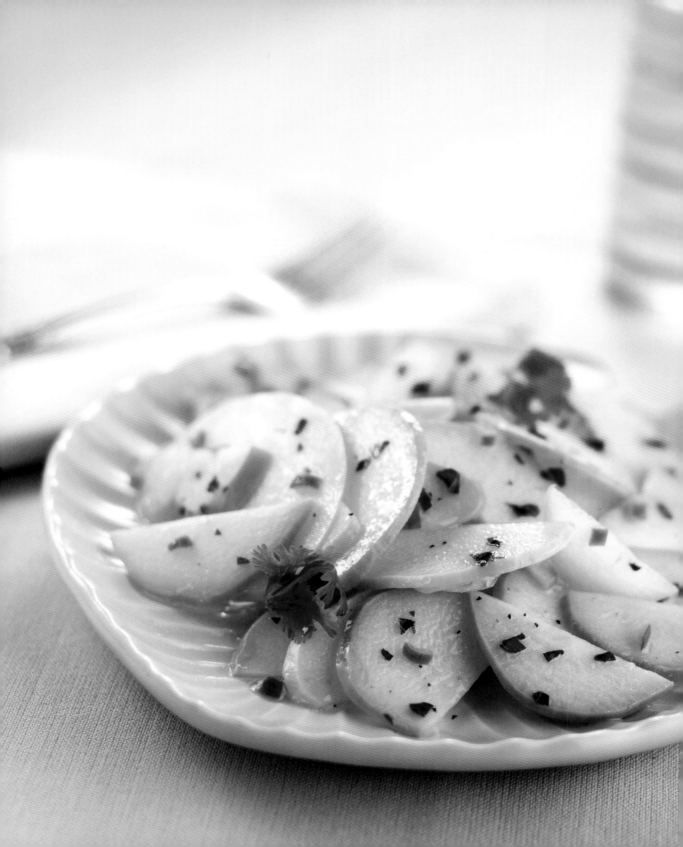

Chayote Salad

The chayote was a favourite fruit of the Aztecs. It goes by many other names, including vegetable pear, mirliton, christophene, chocho and choko. When you are buying chayote, remember that they age much as we do, so if they're wrinkled, they're old. When young, chayote skin is tender and quite edible. If your chayote are not as young as you'd like, peel away the skin before you slice them.

Look for chayote in West Indian shops and markets, but if you can't find them, try this recipe with courgettes (zucchini).

3	chayote, seeded and thinly sliced
1	serrano or jalapeño (hot green) chilli, seeded and finely chopped (wear rubber gloves when handling)
4	tablespoons chopped fresh coriander
	juice of 1 small lemon, strained
80 ml (3 fl oz)	extra virgin olive oil
2	tablespoons cider vinegar
	salt
	freshly ground black pepper
	small sprigs of coriander, to garnish

In a large bowl, combine the chayote, chilli, coriander, lemon juice, oil and vinegar. Toss to coat well. Sprinkle with salt and pepper and garnish with sprigs of coriander.

Makes 4 servings

NUTRITION AT A GLANCE
Per serving: Energy 190 cals/795 kJ; 20 g fat (of which 3 g saturates), 1 g protein, 1 g carbohydrate (of which 1 g sugars), 0.5 g fibre, 196 mg sodium

Couscous Salad

Here's a fresh-tasting salad that's perfect for a light lunch.

90 g (3 oz)	couscous
240 ml (8 fl oz)	boiling chicken stock
2	tablespoons extra virgin olive oil
1	tablespoon balsamic vinegar
⅛	teaspoon salt
¼	teaspoon ground black pepper
1	tomato, seeded and finely chopped
1	small cucumber, peeled and finely chopped
90 g (3 oz)	feta cheese, crumbled
285 g (10 oz)	baby spinach leaves, stems removed

In a large bowl, combine the couscous and the boiling stock. Stir well, then cover and set aside for 5 minutes, or until the liquid is absorbed.

Meanwhile, whisk together the olive oil, balsamic vinegar, salt and pepper. Add to the couscous, along with the tomato and cucumber and toss until blended. Cover and refrigerate until ready to serve.

Just before serving, add the cheese and most of the spinach to the couscous and toss. Line a serving platter with the remaining spinach leaves and spoon the couscous mixture on top.

Makes 4 servings

NUTRITION AT A GLANCE
Per serving: Energy 182 cals/762 kJ; 6 g fat (of which 3 g saturates), 11 g protein, 22 g carbohydrate (of which 5 g sugars), 3 g fibre, 892 mg sodium

Overnight Coleslaw

If you're looking for a delicious way to boost your fibre intake, it's hard to beat an old-fashioned cabbage salad.

2–4	tablespoons sugar substitute
4	tablespoons lemon juice
4	tablespoons white vinegar
1	teaspoon celery salt
1	teaspoon garlic salt
1	small head white cabbage, shredded
3	sticks of celery, chopped
½	green pepper (capsicum), chopped
4	tablespoons chopped fresh chives
30 g (1 oz)	radishes, sliced

In a large bowl, whisk together 2 tablespoons of the sugar substitute, the lemon juice, vinegar, celery salt and garlic salt. Taste and add more sugar substitute if you like. Add the cabbage, celery, green pepper and chives and toss lightly. Cover and refrigerate overnight.

Add the radishes immediately before serving.

Makes 4 servings

NUTRITION AT A GLANCE
Per serving: Energy 50 cals/209 kJ; 0.5 g fat (of which 0 g saturates), 2 g protein, 8 g carbohydrate (of which 7 g sugars), 3 g fibre, 1000 mg sodium

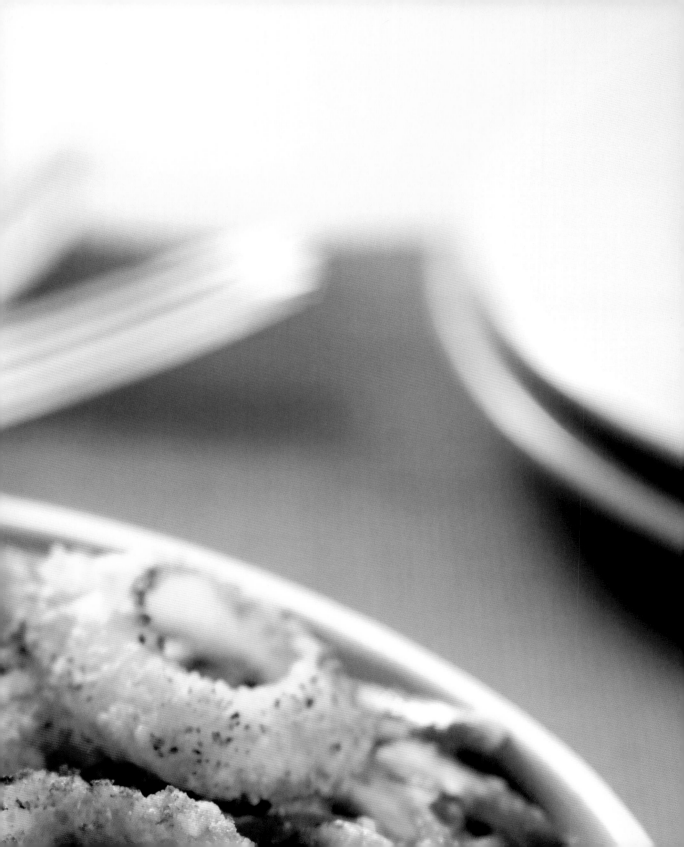

SIDE DISHES AND ACCOMPANIMENTS

SIDE DISHES CAN BE DIVIDED INTO TWO MAIN GROUPS: THE ABSOLUTELY HEALTHY KIND (VEGETABLES, FOR THE MOST PART, ESPECIALLY GREEN ONES) AND THE KIND THAT SUPPLY STARCHES AND CARBS, SUCH AS POTATOES, RICE, PASTA, DUMPLINGS AND THE REST. IDEALLY, PEOPLE ON THE SOUTH BEACH DIET WILL RELY HEAVILY ON THE HEALTHY VEGETABLES. TO ASSIST IN THAT EFFORT, WE'VE DEVISED SOME NEW, TASTY WAYS TO PREPARE THEM, METHODS THAT TURN OUT COLOURFUL, MEMORABLE DISHES WITHOUT ADDING ANY UNNECESSARY STARCHES.

IN THIS CHAPTER, YOU'LL ALSO FIND RECIPES FOR SOME DELICIOUS SAUCES AND DRESSINGS THAT YOU CAN USE TO PERK UP SALADS, VEGETABLES AND SIMPLY COOKED FISH, POULTRY AND MEAT AT EVERY PHASE OF THE SOUTH BEACH DIET.

Edamame with Spring Onions and Sesame

'Edamame' is the Japanese name for green soya beans. These tasty beans have exploded in popularity in recent years; look for them in Japanese, Thai and Chinese food shops. Give them a try, and soon you'll be hooked! The easy cooking method used here has this dish ready in 15 minutes.

340 g (12 oz)	fresh or frozen shelled edamame
1	tablespoon light soy sauce
120 ml (4 fl oz)	water
1½	teaspoons sesame oil
1	teaspoon rapeseed (canola) oil
	dash of Tabasco (optional)
2	tablespoons finely chopped spring onions
⅛	teaspoon ground black pepper

Bring the edamame, soy sauce and water to the boil in a medium saucepan over medium–high heat. Reduce the heat to low and simmer, stirring occasionally, for 12 minutes, or until tender. If any liquid remains, increase the heat and cook, stirring occasionally, until the liquid has evaporated.

Remove from the heat. Stir in the sesame oil, rapeseed oil, Tabasco, if using, spring onions and black pepper.

Makes 4 servings

NUTRITION AT A GLANCE
Per serving: Energy 142 cals/594 kJ; 8 g fat (of which 1 g saturates), 12 g protein, 5 g carbohydrate (of which 2 g sugars), 5 g fibre, 216 mg sodium

Glazed Red Peppers and Mangetouts

A sweet and tangy glaze of balsamic vinegar replaces butter in this spring side dish. If you prefer sugar snap peas, they work well in place of the mangetouts (snow peas).

285 g (10 oz)	mangetouts (snow peas), trimmed
3	tablespoons water
80 ml (3 fl oz)	balsamic vinegar
1	teaspoon sugar substitute
1	teaspoon extra virgin olive oil
2	large red peppers (capsicums), cut into short strips
1	clove garlic, finely chopped
⅛	tablespoon salt
⅛	teaspoon ground black pepper

Place the mangetouts and water in a large microwaveable bowl. Cover with pierced plastic wrap and microwave on high power for a total of 5 minutes, or until crisp-tender; stop and stir after 3 minutes. Drain.

Bring the vinegar and sugar substitute to the boil in a small saucepan over medium-high heat. Cook, stirring constantly, for 3 minutes, or until the mixture is reduced to 2 tablespoons. Remove from the heat.

Warm the oil in a large non-stick frying pan over medium heat. Add the peppers and garlic and cook for 2 minutes, or until crisp-tender. Add the mangetouts, salt, black pepper and the vinegar glaze. Toss to mix.

Makes 4 servings

NUTRITION AT A GLANCE

Per serving: Energy 58 cals/243 kJ; 1 g fat (of which 0 g saturates), 3 g protein, 8 g carbohydrate (of which 7 g sugars), 3 g fibre, 203 mg sodium

Sautéed Peppers and Onions

There's nothing quite so tasty as sautéed peppers (capsicums) and onions, a tender-sweet combination that goes well with just about any main dish. Here the flavour is enhanced with the addition of balsamic vinegar, basil and juicy tomatoes.

1	tablespoon extra virgin olive oil
4	large peppers (capsicums), cut into 5 cm (2 in) wedges
1	large red onion, sliced and separated into rings
1	tablespoon balsamic vinegar
2	tablespoons fresh basil
¼	teaspoon salt
¼	teaspoon ground black pepper
2	plum tomatoes, chopped
3	tablespoons chicken or vegetable stock or water

Heat the oil in a large frying pan over medium heat. Add the peppers and onion and cook, stirring occasionally, for 5 minutes, or until the onion starts to soften.

Add the vinegar, basil, salt and pepper and cook for 1 minute. Add the tomatoes and stock or water. Reduce the heat to low, cover and simmer, stirring occasionally, for 8 minutes, or until the vegetables are very tender.

Makes 4 servings

NUTRITION AT A GLANCE
Per serving: Energy 98 cals/410 kJ; 4 g fat (of which 0.5 g saturates), 3 g protein, 14 g carbohydrate (of which 13 g sugars), 3.5 g fibre, 283 mg sodium

Orange-Ginger Green Beans

Orange and ginger give ordinary green beans a snappy Oriental flavour.

455 g (1 lb)	green beans
1	tablespoon trans-fat-free butter substitute
90 g (3 oz)	shallots, chopped
1	tablespoon finely chopped fresh ginger
½	teaspoon grated orange zest

Bring a saucepan of water to the boil over medium-high heat. Add the beans, cover and simmer for 5 minutes, or until tender. Drain and transfer to a bowl.

Melt the butter substitute in the same pan over low heat. Add the shallots and ginger and sauté for 5 minutes, or until the shallots are tender. Add the beans and orange zest and toss to combine.

Makes 6 servings

NUTRITION AT A GLANCE
Per serving: Energy 48 cals/200 kJ; 3 g fat (of which 0.5 g saturates), 1.5 g protein, 4 g carbohydrate (of which 2 g sugars), 2 g fibre, 27 mg sodium

Green Bean Casserole

This is the South Beach version of a favourite family recipe from the US.

120 ml (4 fl oz)	buttermilk	1	onion, finely chopped
1	slice day-old wholemeal bread	½	teaspoon dried thyme
20 g (¾ oz)	ground walnuts	¼	teaspoon salt
1	onion, cut crosswise into 5-mm (¼-in) thick slices and separated into rings	30 g (1 oz)	wholemeal flour
		700 ml (1¼ pints)	skimmed milk
230 g (8 oz)	portobello or chestnut mushrooms, sliced	455 g (1 lb)	frozen sliced green beans, thawed and drained

Preheat the oven to 120°C/250°F/gas ½. Place the bread on a baking sheet in the oven until dry and crisp. Leave to cool, then crush with a rolling pin or grind to crumbs in a food processor.

Turn up the oven to its highest setting. Coat a baking sheet and a 1.2-litre (2-pint) baking dish with cooking spray.

Place the buttermilk in a shallow bowl. Place the breadcrumbs and walnuts in another shallow bowl; stir to combine. Dip the onion rings into the buttermilk, then dredge in the breadcrumbs and place on the prepared baking sheet. Coat the onion rings lightly with cooking spray. Bake for 20 minutes, or until tender and golden brown.

Meanwhile, coat a saucepan with cooking spray and place over medium heat. Add the mushrooms, chopped onion, thyme and salt. Coat with cooking spray. Cook, stirring occasionally, for 4 minutes, or until the mushrooms release their liquid. Sprinkle with the flour and cook, stirring, for 1 minute. Add the milk and cook, stirring constantly, for 3 minutes, or until thickened. Add the green beans and stir to combine.

Reduce the oven temperature to 200°C/400°F/gas 6. Pour the bean mixture into the prepared baking dish. Scatter the onion rings over the top. Bake for 25 minutes, or until hot and bubbly.

Makes 8 servings

NUTRITION AT A GLANCE
Per serving: Energy 107 cals/448 kJ; 2 g fat (of which 0.5 g saturates), 7 g protein, 15 g carbohydrate (of which 9 g sugars), 2 g fibre, 176 mg sodium

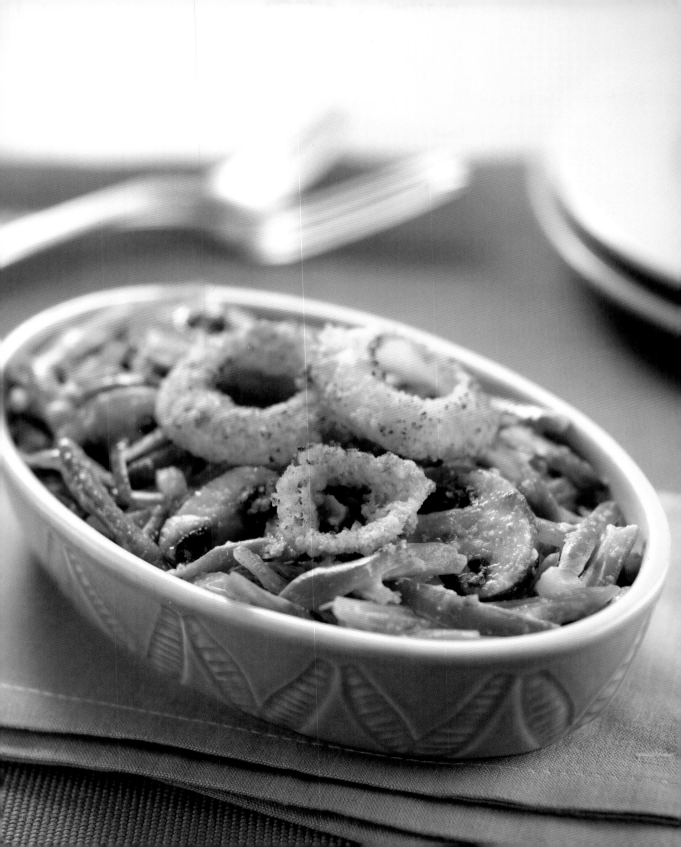

Sesame-Caraway Mixed Vegetables

Even if you think you don't like Brussels sprouts, give them a try in this tasty recipe. Nutty sesame and anise-like caraway add a wonderful flavour accent.

1	tablespoon sesame seeds
2	teaspoons caraway seeds
2	teaspoons extra virgin olive oil
6	spring onions, chopped
250 g (9 oz)	Brussels sprouts, halved
120 ml (4 fl oz)	chicken stock
145 g (5 oz)	mangetouts (snow peas), trimmed
1½	teaspoons ground black pepper
½	teaspoon Italian herb seasoning (low-sodium if available)

Combine the sesame seeds and caraway seeds in a large non-stick frying pan over medium heat. Toast the seeds, shaking the pan often, for 2 minutes, or until fragrant. Transfer to a bowl.

Add the oil to the pan and increase the heat to medium–high. Add the spring onions and stir-fry for 1 minute. Add the Brussels sprouts and stir-fry for 2 minutes. Add the stock, cover and simmer for 5 minutes, or until the vegetables are just tender.

Add the mangetout and cook, stirring often, for 2 minutes, or until the mangetout are crisp-tender. Stir in the seeds, pepper and herb seasoning and cook for 1 minute.

Makes 4 servings

NUTRITION AT A GLANCE
Per serving: Energy 91 cals/380 kJ; 6 g fat (of which 1 g saturates), 5 g protein, 5 g carbohydrate (of which 3.5 g sugars), 4 g fibre, 135 mg sodium

Sesame-Ginger Asparagus

Slender asparagus always makes an elegant side dish. Sprinkled with sesame seeds and with a hint of ginger and chilli, it takes on an Oriental flavour. This is lovely served with a fish main course.

685 g (1½ lb)	thin asparagus, trimmed and cut diagonally into 5 cm (2 in) pieces
1	tablespoon rapeseed (canola) oil
1	tablespoon chopped fresh ginger
1	tablespoon light soy sauce
¼	teaspoon dried chilli flakes
1	teaspoon sesame oil
1	teaspoon sesame seeds

Bring 5 mm (¼ in) water to the boil in a large non-stick frying pan over high heat. Add the asparagus and return to the boil. Reduce the heat to low, cover and simmer for 5 minutes, or until crisp-tender. Drain and cool briefly under cold running water. Wipe the frying pan dry with a paper towel.

Heat the rapeseed oil in the same pan over high heat. Add the asparagus, ginger, soy sauce and chilli flakes and cook for 2 minutes, or until heated through. Remove from the heat and stir in the sesame oil and sesame seeds.

Makes 4 servings

NUTRITION AT A GLANCE
Per serving: Energy 94 cals/393 kJ; 6 g fat (of which 1 g saturates), 6 g protein, 4 g carbohydrate (of which 3 g sugars), 3 g fibre, 217 mg sodium

Fried Green Tomatoes

You don't have to be from the southern States to appreciate this traditional Southern recipe, and these tomatoes aren't fried in the traditional way. Enjoy these as a side dish, or whip up a batch 'just because'.

60 g (2 oz) wholemeal flour

60 g (2 oz) pecan nuts, finely chopped

1½ teaspoons ground black pepper

6 large green tomatoes, cut into 1 cm (½ in) slices

2 tablespoons rapeseed (canola) oil

1 tablespoon chopped fresh basil

In a shallow bowl, combine the flour, pecans and pepper. Dip the tomatoes into the mixture, turning to coat both sides.

Heat the oil in a large, heavy frying pan over medium–high heat. Working in batches, add the tomatoes in a single layer. Reduce the heat to low and cook slowly until they are brown on one side. Turn the tomatoes carefully and cook until the inside is tender and the second side is brown. Remove each slice as it is finished and place on a warm serving dish. Repeat until all the tomatoes are cooked.

Pour the pan juices over the tomatoes and sprinkle with the basil.

Makes 6 servings

NUTRITION AT A GLANCE

Per serving: Energy 151 cals/734 kJ; 11 g fat (of which 1 g saturates), 3 g protein, 10 g carbohydrate (of which 4 g sugars), 2 g fibre, 10 mg sodium

Cheesy Baked Artichokes

Artichokes baked gratin-style are creamy and delicious. Using frozen or tinned hearts makes this recipe a breeze to prepare.

500 g (1 lb 2 oz)	frozen artichoke hearts
	or
2 × 280 g (10 oz)	jars artichoke hearts in olive oil, drained
1	tablespoon lemon juice
3	tablespoons ground pecan nuts
2	tablespoons grated Parmesan cheese
1	teaspoon Italian herb seasoning
1	clove garlic, finely chopped
1	teaspoon extra virgin olive oil

Preheat the oven to 190°C/375°F/gas 5. Coat a baking dish with cooking spray.

Place the artichokes in a colander and rinse well with cold water. Drain well, then pat dry with paper towels. Place in the prepared dish and sprinkle with the lemon juice.

In a small bowl, combine the pecans, cheese, herb seasoning, garlic and oil. Sprinkle the mixture evenly over the artichokes.

Bake for 15 minutes, or until the topping is golden.

Makes 4 servings

NUTRITION AT A GLANCE
Per serving: Energy 190 cals/795 kJ; 13 g fat (of which 3 g saturates), 11 g protein, 7 g carbohydrate (of which 6 g sugars), 4 g fibre, 100 mg sodium

Courgettes with Cheese and Walnuts

Chopped walnuts and Parmesan give this delightful dish a nutty, rich flavour.

2	teaspoons trans-fat-free butter substitute
2	large cloves garlic, finely chopped
2	medium courgettes (zucchini), cut into 8 cm (3 in) sticks
2	medium yellow courgettes (zucchini), cut into 8 cm (3 in) sticks
2	tablespoons chicken or vegetable stock
⅛	teaspoon salt
⅛	teaspoon ground black pepper
30 g (1 oz)	chopped walnuts, toasted
45 g (1½ oz)	Parmesan or aged Asiago cheese, grated

Melt the butter substitute in a large non-stick frying pan over medium-low heat. Add the garlic and cook, stirring constantly, for 1 minute, or until soft.

Add the courgettes, stock, salt and pepper. Bring to a simmer over medium heat. Cover and simmer, stirring occasionally, for 6 minutes, or until the courgettes are tender. Transfer to a warm serving dish and sprinkle with the walnuts and cheese.

Makes 4 servings

NUTRITION AT A GLANCE
Per serving: Energy 150 cals/628 kJ; 11 g fat (of which 3 g saturates), 8 g protein, 4 g carbohydrate (of which 3 g sugars), 1.5 g fibre, 390 mg sodium

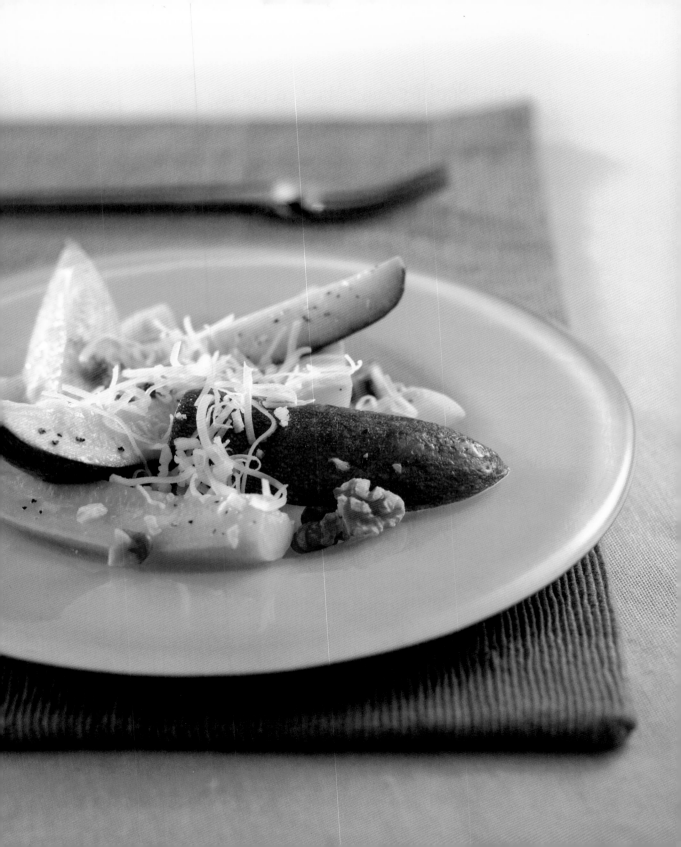

Surprise South Beach 'Mashed Potatoes'

You won't believe how many people you'll fool with this recipe. And think how easy it is to make — you don't have to peel the potatoes!

455 g (1 lb)	cauliflower florets	pinch of salt
30 g (1 oz)	trans-fat-free butter substitute	pinch of ground black pepper
1–2	tablespoons skimmed milk	

Place a steamer basket in a large saucepan over boiling water. Place the cauliflower in the basket and bring to the boil over high heat. Reduce the heat to medium, cover and cook for 4 minutes, or until just tender. Purée in a food processor, adding the butter substitute and the milk. Season with salt and pepper.

Makes 4 servings

NUTRITION AT A GLANCE
Per serving: Energy 97 cals/406 kJ; 7 g fat (of which 1.5 g saturates), 4 g protein, 4 g carbohydrate (of which 3 g sugars), 2 g fibre, 171 mg sodium

Roasted Pepper Cream

The warmth of the peppers (capsicums) merges with the coolness of the yogurt.

200 g (7 oz)	roasted red peppers (capsicums) in olive oil, drained	1 teaspoon cider vinegar
2	tablespoons fat-free natural yogurt or virtually fat-free natural fromage frais	salt
		ground black pepper

In a blender or food processor, combine the peppers, yogurt or fromage frais, vinegar, and salt and pepper to taste. Store in a sealed container in the refrigerator until ready to serve.

Makes about 240 ml (8 fl oz)

NUTRITION AT A GLANCE
Per 2 tablespoons: Energy 20 cals/84 kJ; 1 g fat (of which 0 g saturates), 1 g protein, 2 g carbohydrate (of which 2 g sugars), trace fibre, 102 mg sodium

Aubergine 'Spaghetti' Sauce

I created this sauce to serve with spaghetti squash, but you can use it with any of the vegetables on the acceptable list.

> 1 small aubergine (eggplant), cut lengthwise into 1 cm (½ in) slices
>
> 1 tablespoon extra virgin olive oil
>
> 1 small onion, chopped
>
> 1 clove garlic, finely chopped
>
> 2 × 400 g (14 oz) tins peeled plum tomatoes
>
> 2 tablespoons tomato purée (concentrate)
>
> 2 tablespoons chopped fresh basil

Preheat the grill.

Lightly coat the aubergine slices with olive oil cooking spray. Place on a grill rack and grill until the aubergine slices are brown on both sides. Remove from the heat and cut into 2–3 cm (1 in) pieces.

Heat the oil in a large saucepan over medium heat. Add the onion and garlic and cook for 3 minutes, or until tender. Stir in the tomatoes (with juice), tomato purée and basil. Cook, stirring to break up the tomatoes, for 5 minutes, or until the mixture begins to boil. Reduce the heat to low, partially cover and simmer, stirring occasionally, for 15 minutes. Add the aubergine, stir to combine, and simmer for another 5 minutes.

Makes 4 servings (1.2 litres/2 pints)

NUTRITION AT A GLANCE
Per serving: Energy 82 cals/543 kJ; 3 g fat (of which 0.5 g saturates), 3 g protein, 11 g carbohydrate (of which 9 g sugars), 3 g fibre, 104 mg sodium

South Beach Tomato Sauce

You can use this light sauce in any recipe that calls for a tomato sauce or simply as a topping for chicken or fish.

4	tablespoons extra virgin olive oil
½	onion, finely chopped
2 × 400 g (14 oz)	tins peeled plum tomatoes
60 ml (2 fl oz)	dry white wine
2	cloves garlic, finely chopped
4	leaves fresh basil, chopped
2	tablespoons chopped fresh parsley
½	teaspoon sugar substitute
	pinch of cayenne pepper
30 g (1 oz)	pitted black olives, coarsely chopped

Heat the oil in a saucepan over medium heat. Add the onion and cook, stirring occasionally, for 3 minutes, or until soft. Add the tomatoes (with juice), wine, garlic, basil, parsley, sugar substitute and pepper. Reduce the heat to low and simmer for 1 hour.

Add the olives and simmer for a further 3 minutes. Store in a covered container in the refrigerator until ready to serve.

Makes about 480 ml (16 fl oz)

NUTRITION AT A GLANCE

Per 4 tablespoons: Energy 80 cals/335 kJ; 6 g fat (of which 1 g saturates), 1 g protein, 4 g carbohydrate (of which 3 g sugars), 1 g fibre, 124 mg sodium

From the Menu of . . .

JOE'S STONE CRAB

11 Washington Avenue, Miami Beach, Florida

CHEF ANDRE BIENVENU

FOUNDED IN 1913 AND STILL FAMILY RUN, *JOE'S STONE CRAB* IS AN
EVER-POPULAR MIAMI BEACH PHENOMENON.

Sweet Onion Dressing

PHASE 3

- 1 onion (about 115 g/4 oz), halved
- 8 cloves garlic, chopped
- 4 tablespoons chopped fresh parsley,
- 2 tablespoons sugar
- 8 tablespoons Dijon mustard
- 480 ml (16 fl oz) olive oil
- 60 ml (2 fl oz) white wine vinegar
- 120 ml (4 fl oz) water
- 1 teaspoon sea salt
- 1 teaspoon black pepper

Preheat the grill or preheat the oven to 200°C/400°F/gas 6.
Grill or roast the onion until light brown, about 10 to 15 minutes.
Place the onion in a food processor and pulse until finely chopped.
Add the garlic, parsley, sugar and mustard and process. Slowly add the
oil. Add the vinegar, water, salt and pepper and process until well
combined.

Makes 16 servings (4 tablespoons per serving)

NUTRITION AT A GLANCE
Per 4 tablespoons: Energy 292 cals/1222 kJ; 30 g fat (of which 4 g saturates), 1 g protein,
4 g carbohydrate (of which 3 g sugars), 0 g fibre, 359 mg sodium

South Beach Green Goddess Dressing

A South Beach twist on a classic recipe from the '70s.

115 g (4 oz)	mayonnaise
115 g (4 oz)	fat-free natural yogurt
30 g (1 oz)	anchovy fillets, chopped
4 tablespoons	chopped fresh parsley
3	spring onions, chopped
1	tablespoon white wine vinegar
½	teaspoon salt
⅛	teaspoon garlic powder
⅛	teaspoon ground black pepper

In a small bowl, combine the mayonnaise, yogurt, anchovies, parsley, spring onions, vinegar, salt, garlic powder and pepper and mix well. Store in a covered container in the refrigerator until ready to serve. (Keeps for 1 week.)

Makes about 240 ml (8 fl oz)

NUTRITION AT A GLANCE
Per tablespoon: Energy 60 cals/251 kJ; 6 g fat (of which 1 g saturates), 1 g protein, 1 g carbohydrate (of which 0.5 g sugars), 0 g fibre, 185 mg sodium

Herb Vinaigrette

This tasty vinaigrette is sure to spice up your salads.

120 ml (4 fl oz) white wine vinegar

120 ml (4 fl oz) extra virgin olive oil

2 tablespoons chopped fresh basil

2 tablespoons chopped fresh tarragon

2 tablespoons chopped fresh parsley

2 tablespoons chopped fresh marjoram

2 teaspoons chopped fresh oregano

2 tablespoons drained and chopped capers

1 teaspoon Dijon mustard

½ teaspoon sugar substitute

ground black pepper (optional)

Put all the ingredients into a screw-topped jar, close the lid tightly and shake vigorously. Store in the refrigerator until ready to serve. (Keeps for 1 week.)

Makes 350 ml (12 fl oz)

NUTRITION AT A GLANCE
Per tablespoon: Energy 48 cals/200 kJ; 5 g fat (of which 1 g saturates), 0 g protein, 0 g carbohydrate, 0 g fibre, 17 mg sodium

South Beach Condiments

When watching what you eat, it's easy to forget about what goes *on top* of what you eat. After all, amid the delights of a cheeseburger, fries and soda, how dangerous do a few squirts of ketchup seem? But we ignore these toppings at our own risk, because condiments, dressings and so on can pack their own bad carb punch. This is especially true today, when we're enticed by the endless array of sauces found in supermarkets and restaurants. We've gone way beyond the basic trio of ketchup, mustard and mayo. Young diners who have been raised in the fast-food era would be lost without their dipping sauces – chicken nuggets, for instance, *always* come with a sauce to dunk them into. Many of today's most popular condiments, savoury sauces and toppings are laden with bad carbs in the form of sugar or other sweeteners.

Ketchup, by dint of its popularity, is a prime diet-buster. It isn't meant to sweeten your food, and it does taste mostly of tomato, vinegar and spices. But examine the label: right up there near the top of the list, you'll find glucose syrup/corn syrup and other forms of sugar. In a single serving of 1 tablespoon, there are 4 grams of sugar – that's virtually 1 teaspoon of pure sugar.

Mustard, on the other hand, is a perfectly healthy condiment. It has no carbs or fat to speak of, and it enhances the flavour of food, which is a good objective. Still, there is a way to make mustard hazardous. One of today's most popular varieties is honey mustard, which contains a substantial amount of sugar. Examine the labels and compare: regular mustard has no sugar whatsoever; in honey mustard, you may find sugar, honey and molasses among the ingredients. It's used most often as a dipping sauce and in salad dressings.

Mayonnaise has a bad reputation because of the calories from the fats and oils it contains. But today, most brands use rapeseed (canola) or olive oil, so mayo can now be considered part of a healthy diet. It is a good source of vitamin E, plus it's filling and makes food taste good.

Barbecue sauces usually fall into two categories: savoury (vinegar-based) or sweet (which contain brown sugar, molasses, or glucose syrup/corn syrup). Guess which kind is most popular these days? Hands down, it's the sweet. And even the vinegar-based varieties are often made with sweeteners. Added sugars show up unexpectedly nowadays in everything from brown sauce, which may also contain raisins for sweetness, to seafood cocktail sauce.

As we've noted, honey-based dipping sauces are all the rage these days, thanks to the fast-food influence on our eating habits. This is why fast food is so bad for people trying to lose weight: not only is it full of bad fats, there are bad carbs lurking there, too. As an alternative, look for no-carb, sugar-free honey vinaigrette salad dressing, which is available from several manufacturers.

One obvious solution to the condiment problem is simply to stick with ones without sugar or seek out brands made with sugar substitutes. But you can also make your own. For instance, you can easily make ketchup that tastes good and keeps to the South Beach Diet. For South Beach Ketchup as well as other delicious homemade condiments, see the recipes beginning on page 162.

South Beach Barbecue Sauce

230 g (8 oz)	passata (sieved tomatoes)	2	teaspoons chopped fresh parsley
2	tablespoons white vinegar	¼	teaspoon salt
1	teaspoon Worcestershire sauce	⅛	teaspoon ground black pepper
1	teaspoon mustard powder	⅛	teaspoon garlic powder

In a resealable container, combine the tomato passata, vinegar, Worcestershire sauce, mustard powder, parsley, salt, pepper and garlic powder. Store in the refrigerator until ready to serve. (Keeps for 1 week.)

Makes about 240 ml (8 fl oz)

NUTRITION AT A GLANCE

Per 2 tablespoons: Energy 12 cals/50 kJ; 0 g fat, 1 g protein, 2 g carbohydrate (of which 1.5 g sugars), 0.5 g fibre, 175 mg sodium

South Beach Cocktail Sauce

230 g (8 oz)	passata (sieved tomatoes)	1	teaspoon chopped parsley
1	tablespoon lemon juice	1	teaspoon prepared horseradish
1	teaspoon Worcestershire sauce	⅛	teaspoon garlic powder
½	teaspoon onion salt		

In a large saucepan over medium heat, combine the tomato passata, lemon juice, Worcestershire sauce, onion salt, parsley, horseradish and garlic powder. Simmer for 5 minutes. Place in a resealable container and store in the refrigerator until ready to serve. (Keeps for 1 week.)

Makes 240 ml (8 fl oz)

NUTRITION AT A GLANCE

Per 2 tablespoons: Energy 11 cals/46 kJ; 0 g fat, 1 g protein, 2 g carbohydrate (of which 1.5 g sugars), 0.5 g fibre, 187 mg sodium

South Beach Teriyaki Sauce

120 ml (4 fl oz) light soy sauce

120 ml (4 fl oz) dry sherry

4 tablespoons sugar-free pancake syrup or 2 tbs sugar substitute

4 tablespoons ground arrowroot

3 tablespoons red wine vinegar

4 cloves garlic, crushed

1 teaspoon ground ginger

¼ teaspoon Tabasco

In a food processor, combine the soy sauce, sherry, syrup or sugar substitute, arrowroot, vinegar, garlic, ginger and Tabasco. Purée until smooth. Place in a resealable container and store in the refrigerator until ready to serve. (Keeps for 1 week.)

Makes 350 ml (12 fl oz)

NUTRITION AT A GLANCE

Per 2 tablespoons: Energy 32 cals/134 kJ; 0 g fat, 1 g protein, 4 g carbohydrate (of which 0 g sugars), 0 g fibre, 576 mg sodium

South Beach Ketchup

230 g (8 oz) passata (sieved tomatoes)

170 g (6 oz) tomato purée (concentrate)

2 tablespoons sugar substitute

2 teaspoons onion powder

2 teaspoons light soy sauce

½ teaspoon ground cloves

½ teaspoon ground allspice

1½ tablespoons malt vinegar

In a large saucepan over medium heat, combine the tomato passata, tomato purée, sugar substitute, onion powder, soy sauce, cloves, allspice and vinegar. Simmer for 5 minutes. Place in a resealable container and store in the refrigerator until ready to serve. (Keeps for 1 week.)

Makes about 240 ml (8 fl oz)

NUTRITION AT A GLANCE

Per 2 tablespoons: Energy 25 cals/104 kJ; 0 g fat, 2 g protein, 5 g carbohydrate (of which 4 g sugars), 1 g fibre, 146 mg sodium

South Beach Spiced Mustard

This recipe requires a little bit of effort, but homemade mustard, like so many things, really does taste better than store-bought.

180 ml (6 fl oz)	water
4	tablespoons mustard seeds
6	tablespoons mustard powder
¼	teaspoon dried tarragon
1	tablespoon turmeric
120 ml (4 fl oz)	tarragon vinegar
120 ml (4 fl oz)	dry white wine
1	tablespoon rapeseed (canola) oil
4	tablespoons sugar substitute
2	cloves garlic, finely chopped
¼	teaspoon ground allspice
¼	teaspoon ground cinnamon
¼	teaspoon ground cloves
½	teaspoon ground arrowroot

In a small bowl, combine the water, mustard seeds, mustard powder, tarragon and turmeric.

In a saucepan, combine the vinegar, wine, oil, sugar substitute, garlic, allspice, cinnamon and cloves. Bring to the boil over medium–high heat and simmer for 5 minutes.

In a blender or food processor, combine the mustard and vinegar mixtures and blend for 2 minutes. Return the mixture to the saucepan and heat over a low heat for 5 minutes. Stir in the arrowroot to thicken. Place in a sealable jar and store in the refrigerator until ready to serve. (Keeps for 1 week.)

Makes about 350 ml (12 fl oz)

NUTRITION AT A GLANCE
Per tablespoon: Energy 15 cals/63 kJ; 1 g fat (of which 0 g saturates), 0.5 g protein, 1 g carbohydrate (of which 0.5 g sugars), 0 g fibre, 10 mg sodium

MY SOUTH BEACH DIET

I'M LIVING PROOF OF THE CONNECTION BETWEEN DIABETES, WEIGHT LOSS AND HEART HEALTH.

I have tried every diet out there, both fad and physician-prescribed, and I've always had the same disappointing outcome. Because previous diets did not fit into my normal, everyday life, I would struggle and give up quickly. At the age of 57, I weighed 127 kg (nearly 20 st) and was taking medication and daily insulin shots to control the type 2 diabetes I have had for 10 years, Since starting the South Beach Diet, my health has rapidly improved. A weight loss of 11.5 kg (25 lb)! Feeling more in control of my life is just an added bonus.

Before South Beach, I started a weight-loss support programme with my daughter and did pretty well, losing 3.6 kg (8 lb) in eight or nine weeks, but then I gained 2.5 kg (5 lb) the following two weeks. Talk about disappointment! At this point I started to believe that I was the typical 'hopelessly overweight' person, who would never lose any more than 4.5 kg (10 lb).

That's when I checked the *Prevention.com* Message Forum and became inspired by what people were saying about the South Beach Diet. Just four days after jumping onto the 'Beach', I weighed in and found that I had lost 3.5 kg (nearly 8 lb). I was ecstatic! Three days after that, I had an appointment with my nurse practitioner and I had lost another kilo (nearly 2 pounds)! She then took me off two of my medications and told me that if my blood sugar stayed within normal limits, I could wean myself off the insulin. I floated out of her office that day.

Since starting the diet, I have stayed more or less on Phase 1, adding back fruit but not pasta, bread or rice. It's good to know that I could have some if I wanted, but I like the way I feel without them.

Although I've had a couple of minor setbacks, I plan on continuing just what I'm doing until I get to around 80 kg (12½ st). It really doesn't look that far away or hopeless to me any more.

I still go to the support programme meetings for the personal interaction and accountability, and I also participate in the South Beach discussion forum online. I think emotional support is really essential in any success. We are all educating ourselves about a new way to live, and any words of wisdom are invaluable.

Overall, the actual pounds lost, while significant, are but a tiny measure of the health changes I've actually experienced. I'm living proof of the connection between diabetes and weight – *CHERYL O*.

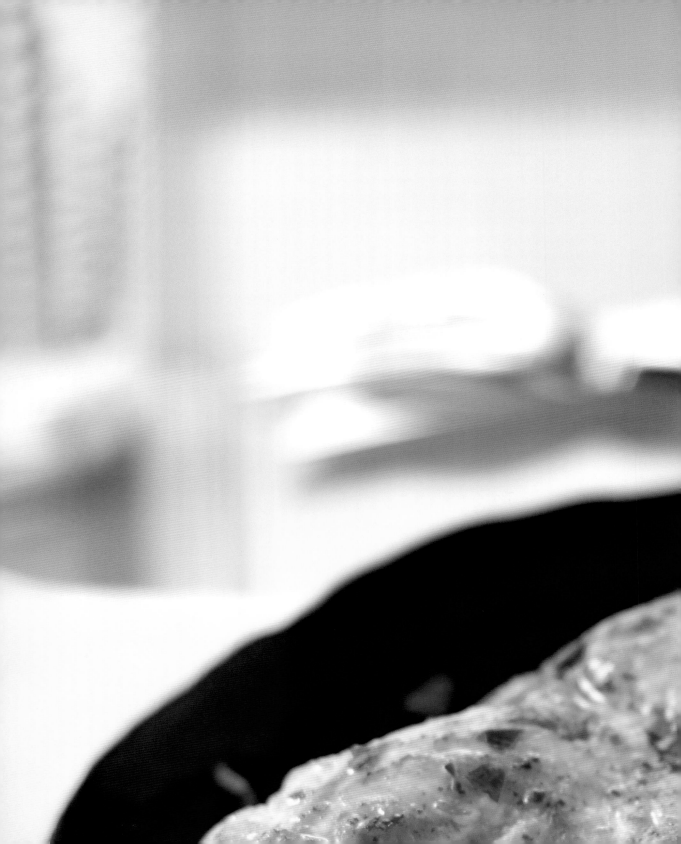

FISH, SHELLFISH AND POULTRY

EATING FISH HAS PRACTICALLY BECOME A FORM OF SELF-MEDICATION, THANKS TO ALL THE NEWS STORIES ABOUT THE HEALTH BENEFITS OF SALMON, TUNA AND THE REST. IT'S ABSOLUTELY TRUE THAT THREE OR FOUR MEALS A WEEK OF THESE SO-CALLED OILY FISH (MACKEREL OR SARDINES, TOO) CAN HELP PREVENT HEART ATTACKS. THE OMEGA-3 FATTY ACIDS THESE FISH CONTAIN KEEP BLOOD PLATELETS FROM FORMING STICKY CLUMPS THAT BLOCK ARTERIES.

SIMILARLY, WE'VE ALL BECOME FAITHFUL FANS OF SKINLESS WHITE-MEAT CHICKEN AND TURKEY FOR REASONS OF WEIGHT CONTROL AND CARDIO-VASCULAR HEALTH. BUT MAKING THESE WISE DIETARY MOVES DOESN'T REQUIRE US TO SACRIFICE ANYTHING WHEN IT COMES TO EATING WELL.

THE SOUTH BEACH DIET REFLECTS ITS FLORIDA ORIGINS ESPECIALLY IN ITS FISH AND SEAFOOD RECIPES. WE'VE ALSO COME UP WITH SOME EXCITING WAYS TO LIFT CHICKEN OUT OF THE ORDINARY, LIKE THE CHICKEN WITH *MOLE* SAUCE, A MEXICAN DISH USING COCOA POWDER.

Zesty Crab Cakes with Creamy Pepper Sauce

Though you can use tinned crabmeat if it's in your cupboard, fresh crabmeat is far superior in these crab cakes. Drizzled with a creamy roasted pepper sauce, this is a recipe you'll make again and again.

Creamy Pepper Sauce

2	roasted red peppers, (capsicums), drained if from a jar
115 g (4 oz)	mayonnaise
	ground black pepper

Crab Cakes

1	teaspoon extra virgin olive oil
½	onion, finely chopped
1	stick of celery, finely chopped
1	egg white
2	tablespoons ground walnuts
2	tablespoons chopped flat-leaved parsley
2	tablespoons mayonnaise
1	tablespoon lemon juice
½	teaspoon ground allspice
½	teaspoon ground ginger
2	teaspoons Worcestershire sauce
½	teaspoon mustard powder
¼	teaspoon celery seeds, crushed
½	teaspoon paprika
455 g (1 lb)	crabmeat, flaked and drained
½	teaspoon Tabasco
45 g (1½ oz)	fresh wholemeal breadcrumbs
	sprigs of flat-leaved parsley, to garnish

To make the sauce: Purée the roasted peppers in a food processor or blender. Add the mayonnaise and black pepper to taste and process briefly to combine. Transfer to a small bowl and store in the refrigerator until ready to use.

To make the crab cakes: Heat the oil in a non-stick frying pan over medium–high heat. Add the onion and celery and cook for 5 minutes, or until soft. Transfer to a large bowl.

Stir in the egg white, walnuts, parsley, mayonnaise, lemon juice, allspice, ginger, Worcestershire sauce, mustard powder, celery seeds and paprika. Blend with a fork. Stir in the crabmeat and Tabasco and mix thoroughly. Form into 8 patties. Place the breadcrumbs in a shallow bowl. Roll the patties in the breadcrumbs to coat completely.

Coat a large non-stick frying pan with cooking spray and place over medium-high heat. Working in batches if necessary, add the crab cakes and cook for 2 minutes. Cover and cook for a further 1 minute, or until browned on the bottom. Coat the tops with cooking spray and turn over. Cook, uncovered, for 2 minutes, or until golden brown. Serve hot, with the sauce dotted on the plates. Garnish with the parsley.

Makes 4 servings

NUTRITION AT A GLANCE
Per serving: Energy 567 cals/2573 kJ; 45 g fat (of which 6 g saturates), 28 g protein, 13 g carbohydrate (of which 7 g sugars), 2.5 g fibre, 864 mg sodium

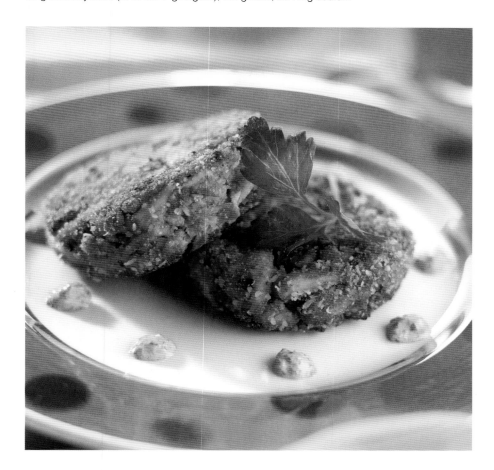

THE LOEWS MIAMI BEACH HOTEL

1601 Collins Avenue, Miami Beach, Florida

EXECUTIVE CHEF MARC EHRLER

THE LOEWS MIAMI BEACH HOTEL, IN THE FABULOUS ART DECO AREA OF SOUTH BEACH, WAS AT THE HEART OF THE MIAMI BEACH RENAISSANCE.

Grilled Fish on Chopped Salad with Olive Oil Lemon Vinaigrette

PHASE 1

1	mahi mahi (dolphinfish), monkfish or swordfish fillet (200 g/7 oz)
	extra virgin olive oil
	salt
	pepper
60 g (2 oz)	iceberg lettuce, torn
20 g (¾ oz)	rocket
1	small cucumber, sliced
90 g (3 oz)	marinated artichokes
½	small red pepper (capsicum), chopped

2	teaspoons finely chopped yellow pepper (capsicum)
30 g (1 oz)	red onion, thinly sliced
1	tablespoon roughly chopped fresh basil
1	tablespoon extra virgin olive oil
2	tablespoons fresh lemon juice

Preheat a ridged grilling pan.

Place the fish on a small plate, drizzle with a little olive oil and season with salt and pepper. Place the fish on the hot grill pan and cook for 2½ minutes. Turn the fish through 45 degrees to create a crisscross pattern and cook for a further 2½ minutes. Flip the fish over and cook in the same way on the other side.

In a mixing bowl, combine the lettuce, rocket, cucumber, artichokes, red pepper, yellow pepper, onion and basil. Toss with the olive oil and lemon juice. Season with salt and pepper to taste. Place the salad on a serving plate and place the cooked fish on top.

Makes 1 serving

NUTRITION AT A GLANCE
Per serving: Energy 469 cals/1963 kJ; 20 g fat (of which 3 g saturates), 50 g protein, 14 g carbohydrate (of which 12 g sugars), 5 g fibre, 500 mg sodium

Ceviche

'Ceviche', 'seviche' and 'cebiche' are all names for the Peruvian/Ecuadorian method of 'cooking' fish by marinating it in lemon or lime juice. Many believe that this delightfully light and simple preparation method was first devised by the Incas.

455 g (1 lb)	monkfish or any firm-fleshed white fresh fish, washed and cut into small cubes
120 ml (4 fl oz)	fresh lime juice
1	clove garlic, crushed
¼–½	teaspoon Tabasco
	salt
	coarsely ground black pepper
1	large onion, finely chopped
1	red pepper (capsicum), cut into strips
1	stick of celery, finely chopped
8	tablespoons chopped fresh coriander

Place the fish in a large glass bowl. Add the lime juice, garlic and Tabasco, and sprinkle with salt and black pepper. Cover and refrigerate for 1 hour.

Add the onion, red pepper, celery and coriander. Cover and refrigerate for a further 1 hour.

Serve chilled in martini glasses for an elegant presentation.

Makes 4 servings

NUTRITION AT A GLANCE
Per serving: Energy 106 cals/443 kJ; 1 g fat (of which 0 g saturates), 20 g protein, 4 g carbohydrate (of which 3 g sugars), 1 g fibre, 384 mg sodium

Crab Royale

While dining on this rich, succulent crab, dim the lights, light the candles and picture yourself in a luxurious restaurant in Paris.

1	slice day-old wholemeal bread, crust removed
230 g (8 oz)	crabmeat, drained and flaked
115 g (4 oz)	reduced-fat Cheddar cheese, grated
4	tablespoons mayonnaise
60 ml (2 fl oz)	skimmed milk
1	stick of celery, finely chopped
2	tablespoons chopped red pepper (capsicum)
2	tablespoons chopped green pepper (capsicum)
1	teaspoon onion powder
1	teaspoon lemon juice
	pinch of black pepper
	pinch of salt

Preheat the oven to 180°C/350°F/gas 4.

Put the bread in a food processor and process to make fine breadcrumbs.

In a large bowl, combine the crabmeat, cheese, breadcrumbs, mayonnaise, milk, celery, red and green pepper, onion, lemon juice, black pepper and salt. Mix thoroughly.

Spoon the mixture into 4 small baking dishes and cook for 15 minutes, or until lightly browned and heated through. Serve hot.

Makes 4 servings

NUTRITION AT A GLANCE
Per serving: Energy 317 cals/1327 kJ; 23 g fat (of which 5 g saturates), 22 g protein, 6 g carbohydrate (of which 2 g sugars), 1 g fibre, 753 mg sodium

From the Menu of . . .

MACALUSO'S

1747 Alton Road, Miami Beach, Florida

CHEF MICHAEL D'ANDREA

THE MENU AT THIS FRIENDLY TRATTORIA IS BASED ON THREE GENERATIONS OF CHEF D'ANDREA'S FAMILY RECIPES, AND EVERYTHING IS HOME-MADE.

Sea Bass Staten Island Style

PHASE 1

3	tablespoons extra virgin olive oil
4	cloves garlic
1	sea bass or other whole, white-fleshed fish (about 285–340 g/10–12 oz), cleaned and scaled
¼	teaspoon salt
¼	teaspoon pepper

½	teaspoon paprika
¼	teaspoon dried chilli flakes
1	teaspoon chopped fresh flat-leaved parsley
½	teaspoon chopped fresh basil
½	lemon

Preheat the oven to 200°C/400°F/gas 6.

In a blender combine the oil and garlic until well blended. Place the fish in a dish, pour the oil mixture over the fish and leave to marinate for about 30 minutes.

Remove the fish from the marinade and place in a small roasting pan, about 2 cm (1 in) larger than the fish. Sprinkle the fish with the salt, pepper, paprika and chilli flakes.

In a small bowl combine the parsley and basil. Sprinkle over the fish. Squeeze the lemon juice over the fish.

Bake the fish for 15 to 20 minutes, or until the fish flakes easily.

Makes 2 servings

NUTRITION AT A GLANCE

Per serving: Energy 278 cals/1163 kJ; 19 g fat (of which 3 g saturates), 24 g protein, 3 g carbohydrate (of which 0.5 g sugars), 0.5 g fibre, 539 mg sodium

Five-Spice Salmon

Chinese five-spice powder is a fragrant blend of fennel, cloves, cinnamon, star anise and Szechuan peppercorns. Orange-Ginger Green Beans (see page 145) are the perfect accompaniment to this spicy salmon.

1½ teaspoons finely grated lime zest	½ teaspoon sugar substitute
3 tablespoons fresh lime juice	4 salmon steaks (about 115 g/4 oz each)
2 teaspoons extra virgin olive oil	285 g (10 oz) fresh baby spinach leaves
4 teaspoons finely chopped fresh ginger	2 cloves garlic, crushed
1 teaspoon Chinese five-spice powder	

In a large dish, combine the lime zest, lime juice, 1 teaspoon of the oil, the ginger, five-spice powder and sugar substitute. Add the salmon and turn to coat. Cover and refrigerate for 30 minutes.

In a large microwaveable dish, combine the spinach, garlic and the remaining 1 teaspoon oil, tossing gently. Cover with plastic wrap and microwave for 2 minutes, or until the spinach has wilted. Drain and keep warm.

Lightly oil a grill rack. Preheat the grill to medium–high.

Remove the salmon from the marinade and place on the grill rack. Brush the salmon with a little of the marinade. Grill for 4 minutes. Turn the salmon, brush with marinade and cook for a further 4 minutes, or until the salmon flakes easily. Discard any remaining marinade.

To serve, divide the spinach among 4 serving plates and place the salmon on top.

Makes 4 servings

NUTRITION AT A GLANCE
Per serving: Energy 247 cals/1034 kJ; 16 g fat (of which 3 g saturates), 24 g protein, 2 g carbohydrate (of which 1.5 g sugars), 2 g fibre, 218 mg sodium

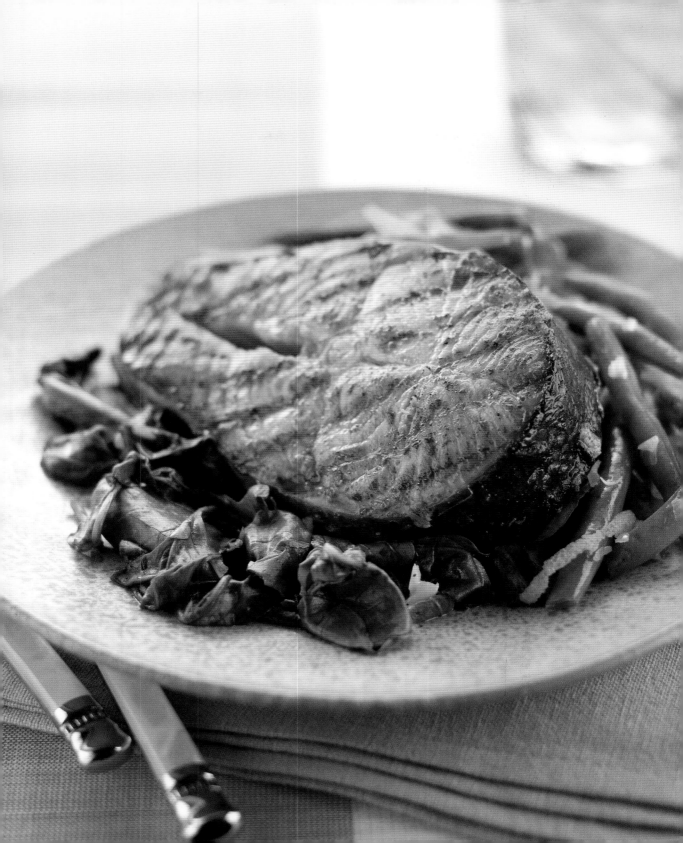

Salmon with Creamy Lemon Sauce

This deceptively simple salmon dish has a sinfully rich-tasting lemony sauce.
For best results, squeeze your own fresh lemon juice.

685 g (1½ lb)	salmon fillet
1	tablespoon extra virgin olive oil
1	clove garlic, finely chopped
4	tablespoons lemon juice
2	tablespoons capers
1	teaspoon lemon-pepper seasoning
120 ml (4 fl oz)	fat-free natural yogurt

Preheat the oven to 180°C/350°F/gas 4. Coat a baking sheet with cooking spray.

Place the salmon on the baking sheet and cook for 20 minutes, or until the fish is just opaque.

Meanwhile, heat the oil in a small saucepan over medium heat. Add the garlic and cook for 1 minute. Reduce the heat to low. Stir in the lemon juice, capers and lemon–pepper seasoning and cook for 5 minutes. Add the yogurt and gently heat through; do not boil. Serve with the fish.

Makes 4 servings

NUTRITION AT A GLANCE
Per serving: Energy 358 cals/1498 kJ; 24 g fat (of which 4 g saturates), 33 g protein, 3 g carbohydrate (of which 3 g sugars), 0.5 g fibre, 279 mg sodium

Pan-Seared Pecan Sea Bass

A coating of wholegrain cereal and pecan nuts gives this fish a wonderful flavour.

3	spring onions, chopped
3	tablespoons South Beach Teriyaki Sauce (see page 163)
1	large clove garlic, finely chopped
1	teaspoon finely chopped fresh ginger
4	fillets of sea bass, snapper or grouper (115 g/4 oz each)
90 g (3 oz)	pecan nuts
20 g (¾ oz)	wholegrain cereal flakes, coarsely crushed
1	teaspoon ground black pepper
2	tablespoons chopped fresh basil

In a shallow glass dish, combine the spring onions, teriyaki sauce, garlic and ginger. Place the fish in the marinade and turn to coat both sides. Cover and refrigerate for 1 to 2 hours.

Meanwhile, toast 30 g (1 oz) of the pecans until fragrant. Leave to cool, then chop. Finely grind the remaining pecans.

In a shallow dish, combine both chopped and ground pecans, crushed cereal and pepper.

Remove the fish from the marinade. Discard the marinade. Press each fillet into the pecan mixture to coat all sides.

Coat a large non-stick frying pan with cooking spray and place over medium–high heat. Add the fish and cook for 3 minutes, or until golden brown on the bottom. Mist the top of the fish with cooking spray, then turn and cook for a further 3 minutes, or until the flesh flakes easily. Sprinkle with the basil and serve hot.

Makes 4 servings

NUTRITION AT A GLANCE
Per serving: Energy 287 cals/1200 kJ; 19 g fat (of which 2 g saturates), 24 g protein, 7 g carbohydrate (of which 2 g sugars), 2 g fibre, 280 mg sodium

From the Menu of . . .

CHINA GRILL

404 Washington Avenue, Miami Beach, Florida

CHEF KEYVAN BEHNAM

CHINA GRILL HAS BEEN A MIAMI HOT SPOT SINCE IT OPENED IN 1995.
IT OFFERS FUNKY 'WORLD FUSION' CUISINE AND FIRST-RATE PEOPLE WATCHING.

Barbecue Salmon

PHASE 3

Salmon

4 ×170 g (6 oz)	salmon fillets, with skin
180 ml (6 fl oz)	barbecue sauce
2	tablespoons rice wine vinegar
2	tablespoons finely chopped spring onions
1	teaspoon finely chopped ginger
	chopped chives, to garnish

Vegetables

½	head Chinese leaves
½	head radicchio
1½	teaspoons extra virgin olive oil

455 g (1 lb)	oyster mushrooms, chopped
120 ml (4 fl oz)	sake or white wine
¼	teaspoon salt
¼	teaspoon pepper

Chinese Mustard Sauce

2	tablespoons mayonnaise
	pinch of mustard powder
⅛	teaspoon Dijon mustard
¾	teaspoon rice wine vinegar
1½	teaspoons finely chopped spring onion

To cook the salmon: Preheat the grill or a ridged grilling pan and coat lightly with cooking spray. Remove the skin of the salmon if desired.

Place the barbecue sauce, vinegar, spring onions and ginger in a blender and mix.

Grill the salmon until cooked to your liking, basting with the barbecue sauce mixture as it cooks. (If you like the skin, cook the skin side first until the skin is crisp, then turn over and baste with the barbecue sauce mixture.)

To cook the vegetables: Remove the hard base of the Chinese leaves and radicchio, then slice the leaves thinly. Heat a sauté pan over high heat. Add the oil and sauté the Chinese leaves, radicchio and mushrooms quickly (they should stay crisp). Add the sake or white wine to the hot pan and stir to coat the vegetables. Add the salt and pepper.

To make the Chinese Mustard Sauce: Place the mayonnaise, mustard powder, mustard, vinegar and spring onion in a blender and mix. Season with salt and pepper to taste.

To serve: Place the sautéed vegetables in the centre of each plate. Dot Chinese Mustard Sauce around the vegetables. Place the salmon on top of the vegetables, sprinkle chopped chives around and serve at once.

Makes 4 servings

NUTRITION AT A GLANCE
Per serving: Energy 472 cals/1975 kJ;
31 g fat (of which 5 g saturates),
35 g protein, 8 g carbohydrate (of
which 2 g sugars), 2 g fibre,
818 mg sodium

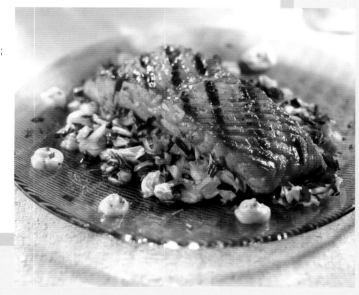

Poached Sea Bass

This is a simple way to prepare a whole fish: use meaty sea bass or another firm-textured fish such as red snapper.

1	sea bass or snapper (230 g/8 oz), cleaned and scaled
60 ml (2 fl oz)	dry white wine
60 ml (2 fl oz)	fish stock or water
1	bay leaf
½	clove garlic, finely chopped
2	plum tomatoes, halved
2	spring onions, chopped
1	sprig of fresh thyme
	pinch of saffron threads

Place the fish in a large non-stick frying pan. Cover with the wine and fish stock and place over medium heat until the liquid begins to shimmer (heat emanates from the liquid). Add the bay leaf, garlic, tomatoes, spring onions, thyme and saffron. Cover and poach for 10 minutes.

Transfer the fish to a serving plate and spoon over the poaching liquid, discarding the bay leaf. Surround with the tomatoes and spring onions.

Makes 2 servings

NUTRITION AT A GLANCE
Per serving: Energy 146 cals/611 kJ; 3 g fat (of which 0.5 g saturates), 22 g protein, 4 g carbohydrate (of which 3.5 g sugars), 1 g fibre, 149 mg sodium

Bombay-Style Sole

Bombay-style cooking is noted for its creamy sauces and the pungent fragrance of its spices. You can also use this marinade for boneless, skinless chicken breasts — just increase the cooking time to 20 minutes.

230 g (8 oz)	fat-free natural yogurt
1	teaspoon curry powder
1	teaspoon ground cardamom
1	teaspoon ground paprika
1	teaspoon ground coriander
4 × 170 g (6 oz)	fillets of sole, skinned
	salt
	ground black pepper

In a small bowl, whisk the yogurt, curry powder, cardamom, paprika and coriander until blended.

Place the sole in a baking dish. Cover with the yogurt mixture. Cover and refrigerate for 2 to 3 hours, turning the fillets about every 30 minutes.

Preheat the oven to 180°C/350°F/gas 4. Cook the sole for 10 minutes, or until it flakes easily. Season with salt and pepper to taste.

Makes 4 servings

NUTRITION AT A GLANCE
Per serving: Energy 181 cals/757 kJ; 4 g fat (of which 1 g saturates), 32 g protein, 6 g carbohydrate (of which 4 g sugars), 0.5 g fibre, 410 mg sodium

Florida Red Snapper

Here's a tasty way to bake a whole fish. Serve with a crisp salad such as Overnight Coleslaw (see page 139).

1 whole red snapper or sea bass (about 900 g/2 lb), cleaned and scaled	1 spring onion, chopped
	60 g (2 oz) pine nuts, toasted
3 tablespoons extra virgin olive oil	2 tablespoons finely chopped fresh parsley
⅛ teaspoon salt	2 tablespoons coarsely chopped almonds, toasted
⅛ teaspoon ground black pepper	3 thin tomato slices
¼ onion, finely chopped	3 thin onion slices
4 tablespoons finely chopped celery	3 thin lime slices
4 tablespoons finely chopped green pepper (capsicum)	juice of ¼ lime

Preheat the oven to 180°C/350°F/gas 4.

Rub the fish lightly with 1 tablespoon of the oil and sprinkle inside and outside with the salt and black pepper.

Heat the remaining 2 tablespoons oil in a small saucepan. Add the chopped onion, celery, green pepper and spring onion and cook, stirring occasionally, for 3 minutes, or until the onion is soft. Stir in the pine nuts, parsley and almonds.

Stuff the fish with the pine nut mixture and tie with kitchen string. Coat a large piece of foil with cooking spray. Place the fish on the foil and cover with alternating overlapping slices of tomato, onion and lime. Sprinkle with salt and black pepper and drizzle with the lime juice. Bring up the edges of the foil and seal. Cook for 30 minutes, or until the fish flakes easily.

Makes 4 servings

NUTRITION AT A GLANCE

Per serving: Energy 434 cals/1816 kJ; 20 g fat (of which 3 g saturates), 40 g protein, 3 g carbohydrate (of which 3 g sugars), 1 g fibre, 336 mg sodium

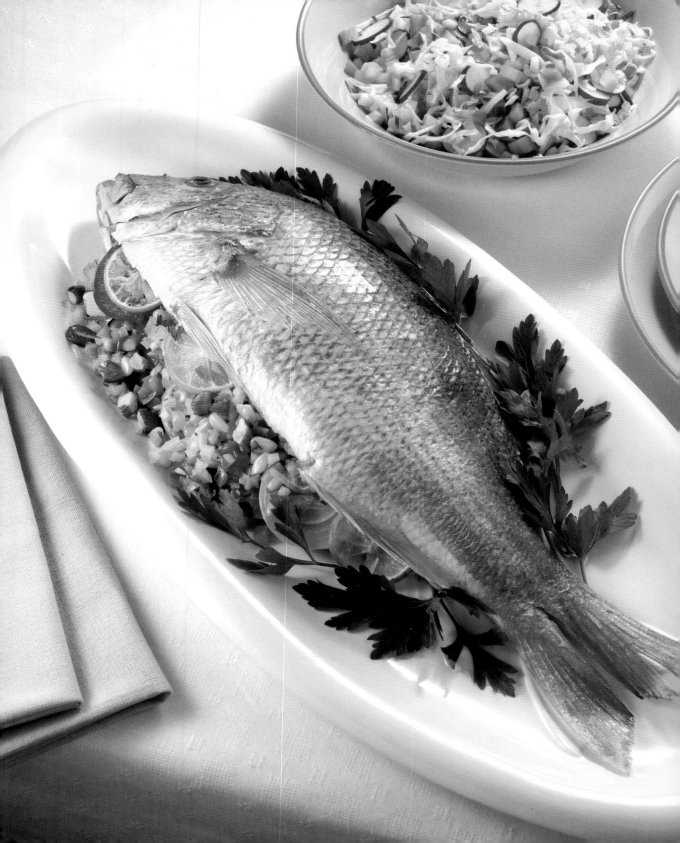

Red Snapper with Avocado Salsa

A cool fish dish for a summer day. See the Vegetarian Chilli with Avocado Salsa (page 288) for the ingredients and preparation of the Avocado Salsa.

500 ml (18 fl oz) water

1 onion, sliced and separated into rings

¼ lime, sliced

1 clove garlic, crushed

2 tablespoons chopped fresh parsley

4 black peppercorns, crushed

½ teaspoon dried thyme, crushed

½ teaspoon dried oregano, crushed

1 whole red snapper, (about 900 g/2 lb), cleaned and scaled

1 teaspoon salt

1 lemon, quartered

1 lime, quartered

sprigs of parsley, to garnish

In a fish poacher or a large shallow pan, combine the water, onion, sliced lime, garlic, parsley, peppercorns, thyme and oregano. Bring to the boil over medium–high heat, then reduce the heat to low, cover and simmer for 5 minutes.

Lightly sprinkle the fish cavity with the salt. Place the fish on a piece of cheesecloth, folding the cloth over the fish. Place on a rack in the poaching pan and immerse in the simmering liquid. If there is not enough liquid to cover the fish, add more boiling water. Cover and poach the fish for 30 minutes, or until the fish flakes easily. Transfer the fish to a serving platter and cover with foil. Refrigerate until cool.

To serve, lift the fillets of fish and discard the bones. Arrange the lemon and lime quarters around the fish fillets and serve with Avocado Salsa. Garnish with the parsley.

Makes 4 servings

NUTRITION AT A GLANCE
Per serving: Energy 218 cals/912 kJ; 4 g fat (of which 1 g saturates), 36 g protein, 4 g carbohydrate (of which 3 g sugars), 0.5 g fibre, 715 mg sodium

Tangy Tuna with Fruit Skewers

Kebabs are always a hit at any barbecue. Here, tangy fruits are combined with juicy cherry tomatoes on skewers to accompany succulent marinated tuna. What a great reason to fire up the barbie!

230 g (8 oz)	tinned pineapple chunks in juice
2	tablespoons light soy sauce
1	teaspoon sesame oil
2	teaspoons finely chopped fresh ginger
¼	teaspoon crushed dried chilli flakes
1	clove garlic, finely chopped
4	tuna steaks (2–3 cm/¾–1 in thick, 145 g/5 oz each)
1	orange, peeled and cut into 8 pieces
4	cherry tomatoes

Drain the juice from the pineapple into a measuring jug and set the chunks aside. Add enough water to the pineapple juice to make 180 ml (6 fl oz). Add the soy sauce, oil, ginger, chilli flakes and garlic and stir to combine. Set aside 2 tablespoons of the liquid. Put the tuna in a sealable plastic bag, add the pineapple juice mixture and seal the bag. Shake well to coat the fish. Refrigerate for at least 30 minutes.

Coat a grill rack with cooking spray. Preheat the grill to medium.

Thread the pineapple chunks, orange pieces and cherry tomatoes on 4 skewers.

Place the fish on the prepared grill rack and cook, brushing with its marinade, for 5 minutes on each side, or until the fish flakes easily.

During the last 3 minutes of cooking, place the fruit skewers on the grill, turning and brushing them with the reserved marinade, for 3 minutes, or until hot.

Makes 4 servings

NUTRITION AT A GLANCE
Per serving: Energy 189 cals/791 kJ; 4 g fat (of which 0.5 g saturates), 27 g protein, 11 g carbohydrate (of which 10 g sugars), 1 g fibre, 554 mg sodium

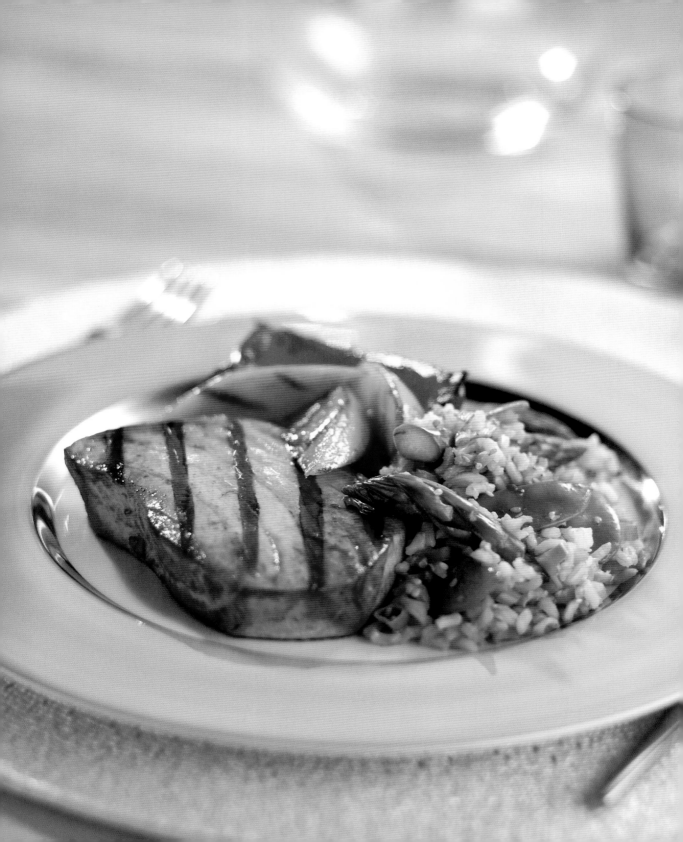

Grilled Tuna with Teriyaki Glaze

This tuna will make your mouth water. Grilled to perfection and brushed with a sassy teriyaki glaze, this is a recipe to satisfy the whole family. Serve with Sesame Mangetout and Asparagus Salad (see page 130) or grilled vegetables.

- 4 tablespoons light soy sauce
- 3 tablespoons dry sherry or chicken stock
- 1 tablespoon grated fresh ginger
- 3 cloves garlic, finely chopped
- 4 tuna steaks (145 g/5 oz each)
- 1 large mango, peeled and cut into spears
- 1 red pepper (capsicum), quartered lengthwise

In a small bowl, combine the soy sauce, sherry or stock, ginger and garlic. Divide the marinade into 2 shallow bowls. Place the tuna in one bowl and the mango and pepper in the other. Turn the tuna, mango and pepper to coat both sides. Cover and refrigerate for 15 minutes.

Coat a grill rack or ridged grilling pan with cooking spray. Preheat the grill to medium or place the pan over medium–high heat.

Place the tuna, mango and pepper on the prepared rack or pan. Discard the marinade from the tuna bowl. Grill, basting occasionally with the marinade from the mango bowl, for 4 minutes on each side, or until the tuna is just opaque and the mango and pepper are heated through and glazed.

Makes 4 servings

NUTRITION AT A GLANCE
Per serving: Energy 250 cals/1046 kJ; 4 g fat (of which 1 g saturates), 36 g protein, 12 g carbohydrate (of which 9 g sugars), 2 g fibre, 990 mg sodium

BARTON G THE RESTAURANT

1427 West Avenue, Miami Beach, Florida

CHEF TED MENDEZ

In 2003, *Condé Nast Traveler* magazine named *Barton G The Restaurant* one of the 75 Top New Restaurants from Boston to Beijing.

Shellfish in a Pot

PHASE 3

2	tablespoons extra virgin olive oil		12	prawns
1	sprig of thyme, chopped		4	extra-large prawns or langoustines
1	bay leaf		20 g (¾ oz)	basil, chopped
2	carrots, chopped		5	baby courgettes (zucchini), sliced
2	sticks of celery, chopped		90 g (3 oz)	leek, cut into matchsticks
1	large onion, chopped		90 g (3 oz)	fennel, cut into matchsticks
2	small shallots, sliced			
3	artichoke bottoms		1	tablespoon pickling spice
3	tablespoons trans-fat-free butter substitute or butter		500 ml (18 fl oz)	shellfish stock (made from boiled shellfish shells)
170 g (6 oz)	green beans, cut diagonally and blanched		4	sprigs of basil
2	small lobster tails, split (170 g/6 oz each)			juice of 1 lemon

Heat the oil in a saucepan, add the thyme, bay leaf, carrots, celery, onion, shallots and artichokes and cook over low heat until lightly browned and caramelized. Add 1 tablespoon of the butter (or substitute) and continue to cook for 25 to 35 minutes or until the artichokes are tender. Remove the artichokes and cut into small wedges. Strain the cooking liquid and reserve.

Reheat the cooking liquid in a casserole. Add the beans and heat for 2 minutes. Stir in the remaining 2 tablespoons of butter (or substitute) and add the lobster, prawns or langoustines and chopped basil. Cover tightly and simmer for 6 to 8 minutes. Remove from the heat and keep covered for a further 4 minutes.

Place the courgettes, leek and fennel in a steamer basket. Add the pickling spice. Steam the vegetables over the shellfish stock until tender, about 3 to 5 minutes. Divide the steamed vegetables and artichokes between 4 soup bowls. Uncover the shellfish and arrange the shellfish and beans on the vegetables. Add the basil sprigs and sprinkle with lemon juice.

Makes 4 servings

NUTRITION AT A GLANCE
Per serving: Energy 280 cals/1172 kJ; 17 g fat (of which 3 g saturates), 21 g protein, 10 g carbohydrate (of which 8 g sugars), 4 g fibre, 1224 mg sodium

Almond Trout Sauté

This sautéed trout goes well with the wonderfully nutty flavour of almonds.

240 ml (8 fl oz)	skimmed milk
1	egg, beaten
100 g (3½ oz)	mushrooms, sliced
50 g (1¾ oz)	hickory smoke-flavoured almonds, chopped
6	tablespoons extra virgin olive oil
2	tablespoons chopped fresh parsley
1	tablespoon lemon juice
4	trout or perch fillets (230 g/8 oz each)

In a small bowl, whisk together the milk and egg. In a large bowl, combine the mushrooms, almonds, 3 tablespoons of the oil, the parsley and lemon juice.

Preheat the oven to 200°C/400°F/gas 6.

Heat the remaining oil in a large non-stick frying pan over medium heat.

Dip the fish in the egg mixture, then place in the frying pan and cook for 3 to 5 minutes, or until golden brown. Turn the fish, place in a non-stick baking dish and place in the oven for 5 minutes.

Meanwhile, wipe the frying pan clean, then add the almond mixture and cook, stirring frequently, for 5 minutes.

To serve, place the fish on a serving platter and spoon the almond mixture over the fish.

Makes 4 servings

NUTRITION AT A GLANCE
Per serving: Energy 420 cals/1758 kJ; 29 g fat (of which 4 g saturates), 40 g protein, 2 g carbohydrate (of which 2 g sugars), 1 g fibre, 168 mg sodium

Cod with Peppercorns and Leeks

Cracked pepper gives a nice bite to mild cod fillets, while leeks sautéed with garlic and lemon are the perfect accompaniment.

½	teaspoon black peppercorns, freshly cracked
½	teaspoon fennel seeds, finely crushed
4	cod, ocean perch or other firm white-fleshed fish fillets (145 g/5 oz each)
1	tablespoon extra virgin olive oil
3	medium leeks, white part only, thinly sliced
3	spring onions, finely chopped
2	cloves garlic, finely chopped
2	teaspoons wholemeal flour
60 ml (2 fl oz)	white wine
60 ml (2 fl oz)	chicken stock
2	tablespoons skimmed milk
½	teaspoon salt

Heat the oven to 190°C/375°F/gas 5.

Press the peppercorns and fennel seeds into both sides of the fish fillets. Set aside.

Heat the oil in an ovenproof frying pan over medium heat. Add the leeks, spring onions and garlic and cook, stirring frequently, for 4 minutes, or until tender. Stir in the flour and cook for 1 minute. Stir in the wine, stock and milk and bring to the boil. Remove from the heat and season with the salt.

Place the fish on top of the leek mixture in the frying pan and bake in the oven for 10 minutes, or until the fish flakes easily.

Makes 4 servings

NUTRITION AT A GLANCE
Per serving: Energy 188 cals/787 kJ; 4 g fat (of which 0.5 g saturates), 28 g protein, 7 g carbohydrate (of which 2.5 g sugars), 2 g fibre, 197 mg sodium

LE BERNARDIN IS NEW YORK CITY'S FINEST SEAFOOD RESTAURANT AND RENOWNED CHEF ERIC RIPERT IS A PARTICIPANT IN FLORIDA'S ANNUAL SOUTH BEACH WINE AND FOOD FESTIVAL.

Sea Bass with Baby Pak Choi and Soy-Ginger Vinaigrette

PHASE 3

12	heads baby pak choi (bok choy), about 900 g/2 lb		small pinch of cayenne pepper
	salt	4	tablespoons water
1	tablespoon finely diced ginger	2	tablespoons unsalted butter
2	tablespoons finely diced shallots		fine sea salt
1	tablespoon oyster sauce		freshly ground white pepper
2	tablespoons sherry vinegar	4	sea bass, grouper or red snapper fillets (200 g/7 oz each)
6	tablespoons rapeseed (canola) oil		
1	tablespoon light soy sauce	1	tablespoon toasted sesame seeds
½	teaspoon fresh lime juice		

Bring a large saucepan of water to the boil. Trim off the root ends of the pak choi, separate the leaves and wash them well. Salt the boiling water and add the pak choi. Blanch until just tender, about 1½ minutes. Immediately plunge the pak choi into a bowl of iced water until cool. Drain and set aside.

Put the ginger and shallots in a mixing bowl and whisk in the oyster sauce and vinegar. Whisk in 4 tablespoons of the oil, the soy sauce, lime juice and cayenne pepper. Set aside.

Bring 4 tablespoons of water to the boil in a large saucepan over high heat. Whisk in the butter and reduce the heat to medium–high. Season the pak choi with salt and pepper, add it to the pan and cook until heated through, about 2 minutes.

Meanwhile, divide the remaining 2 tablespoons of oil between two 25 cm/10 in non-stick frying pans. Place over high heat until the oil is just smoking. Season both sides of the fish with salt and pepper. Place 2 fillets in each pan and sauté until the fish is browned on the bottom, about 3 minutes. Turn and sauté for about 3 minutes on the other side, until the fish flakes easily with a fork.

Lift the pak choi out of the pan with a slotted spoon and arrange it in the centre of 4 dinner plates. Place the fish on top. Whisk the sauce lightly and spoon it around the pak choi. Sprinkle the sesame seeds over the sauce and serve immediately.

Makes 4 servings

NUTRITION AT A GLANCE

Per serving: Energy 472 cals/1975 kJ; 30 g fat (of which 6 g saturates), 41 g protein, 10 g carbohydrate (of which 9 g sugars), 6 g fibre, 958 mg sodium

Seafood-Stuffed Sole

Don't be put off by the number of ingredients here. This elegant dish is quick to assemble and can easily be prepared ahead.

Stuffed Sole

1	teaspoon extra virgin olive oil
2	cloves garlic, finely chopped
60 g (2 oz)	fennel, chopped
4	spring onions, chopped
2	tablespoons chopped flat-leaved parsley
2	tablespoons chopped fresh basil
3	tablespoons chopped shallots
230 g (8 oz)	large prawns, peeled, de-veined and sliced into thirds
115 g (4 oz)	small scallops
45 g (1½ oz)	fresh wholemeal breadcrumbs
1	egg, beaten
1	tablespoon lemon juice
	ground black pepper
4	sole fillets (170 g/6 oz each), skinned
240 ml (8 fl oz)	white wine

Saffron Sauce

1	teaspoon extra virgin olive oil
1	clove garlic, finely chopped
⅛	teaspoon saffron threads, crushed
2	tablespoons hot water
½	teaspoon Dijon mustard
½	teaspoon capers, rinsed and drained
1	tablespoon fat-free natural yogurt
	salt
	ground black pepper
1	tablespoon chopped flat-leaved parsley (optional)

To make the stuffed sole: Preheat the oven to 200°C/400°F/gas 6.

Heat the oil in a large non-stick frying pan over medium heat. Add the garlic, fennel, spring onions, parsley, basil and 2 tablespoons of the shallots. Cook for 4 minutes, or until the fennel is just tender. Add the prawns and scallops and cook for 2 minutes, or until the prawns and scallops are opaque and cooked through.

Transfer the mixture to a large bowl and stir in the breadcrumbs, egg and lemon juice. Season with pepper.

Place the sole, skinned side up, on a work surface. Divide the stuffing into 4 equal portions. Slightly mound the stuffing in the centre of each fillet and roll up the fillets Swiss-roll style.

Coat a 1-litre (2-pint) baking dish with cooking spray. Sprinkle the dish with the remaining 1 tablespoon shallots and place the fillets, seam sides down, on top of the shallots. Pour the wine around the fillets. Cover with a piece of greaseproof paper and cook in the oven for 15 minutes, or until the fish is opaque and flakes easily. Remove from the baking dish and keep warm on a covered serving platter. Reserve the cooking liquid.

To make the saffron sauce: Heat the oil in a small non-stick frying pan over medium heat. Add the garlic and cook for 1 minute. In a cup, mix the saffron with the water and add to the pan. Stir in the mustard, capers and the reserved fish-cooking liquid. Simmer until the liquid is reduced to about 150 ml (5 fl oz). Remove from the heat and whisk in the yogurt. Season with the salt and pepper. Spoon the sauce over the fillets and sprinkle with the parsley, if using.

Makes 4 servings

NUTRITION AT A GLANCE
Per serving: Energy 339 cals/1419 kJ; 7 g fat (of which 1 g saturates), 51 g protein, 8 g carbohydrate (of which 2 g sugars), 1 g fibre, 500 mg sodium

SMITH & WOLLENSKY

1 Washington Avenue, Miami Beach, Florida

CHEF ROBERT MIGNOLA

Smith & Wollensky IS KNOWN AS A GREAT STEAKHOUSE ACROSS THE USA, BUT THIS FIRST-COURSE SALAD SHOWS THERE'S SOMETHING FOR EVERYONE ON THE MENU.

Asparagus, Crab and Grapefruit Salad

PHASE 2

Salad

12	large asparagus spears, trimmed and peeled 8 cm (3 in) at the base of each spear, steamed until just cooked, but still bright green and crisp, then chilled
115 g (4 oz)	mixed salad leaves
230 g (8 oz)	fresh crabmeat, picked over for bits of shell
12	grapefruit segments
1	red pepper (capsicum), chopped
2	tablespoons finely chopped fresh chives

Citrus Vinaigrette

1	teaspoon Dijon mustard
1	tablespoon lemon juice
1	tablespoon lime juice
1	tablespoon orange juice
80 ml (3 fl oz)	extra virgin olive oil
	salt
	pepper

To make the citrus vinaigrette: In a small glass or stainless steel bowl, combine the mustard, lemon juice, lime juice and orange juice. Slowly whisk in the oil. Season with salt and pepper to taste.

To make the salad: Lay 3 asparagus spears on each plate.

Divide the salad leaves into 4 and pile on top of the asparagus to make a bed for the crabmeat. Divide the crabmeat into 4 portions and place it on top of the salad leaves. Arrange the grapefruit segments around the crabmeat. Sprinkle with the red pepper.

Drizzle with citrus vinaigrette and sprinkle with chives.

Makes 4 servings

NUTRITION AT A GLANCE
Per serving: Energy 306 cals/1280 kJ; 23 g fat (of which 3 g saturates), 14 g protein, 10 g carbohydrate (of which 9 g sugars), 3 g fibre, 450 mg sodium

Prawn Creole

Here's a quick way to enjoy the traditional Louisiana dish of shrimp Creole. Serve with hot brown rice for a Phase 2 dinner. If you like, you can substitute scallops for the prawns.

2	rashers turkey bacon or lean back bacon
1	tablespoon extra virgin olive oil (optional)
1	onion, chopped
½	green pepper (capsicum), chopped
1	stick of celery, chopped
1	clove garlic, finely chopped
400 g (14 oz)	tinned chopped tomatoes
1	bay leaf
½	teaspoon ground black pepper
1	teaspoon Worcestershire sauce
1	teaspoon Tabasco
455 g (1 lb)	uncooked prawns, peeled and de-veined

Cook the bacon in a large non-stick frying pan over medium heat until crisp. Place on a paper-towel-lined plate to drain. Crumble when cool. Discard all but 1 tablespoon of the bacon fat from the frying pan; if there is not enough fat, add 1 tablespoon olive oil and heat.

In the hot fat over medium heat, cook the onion, green pepper and celery for 5 minutes, or until tender. Stir in the garlic and cook for 1 minute. Add the tomatoes (with juice), bay leaf, black pepper, Worcestershire sauce and Tabasco. Bring to the boil, then reduce the heat to low and simmer for 20 minutes. Add the prawns and bacon and cook for 5 to 10 minutes, or until the prawns are opaque. Remove and discard the bay leaf before serving.

Makes 4 servings

NUTRITION AT A GLANCE
Per serving: Energy 201 cals/841 kJ; 6 g fat (of which 1 g saturates), 30 g protein, 7 g carbohydrate (of which 5 g sugars), 2 g fibre, 1000 mg sodium

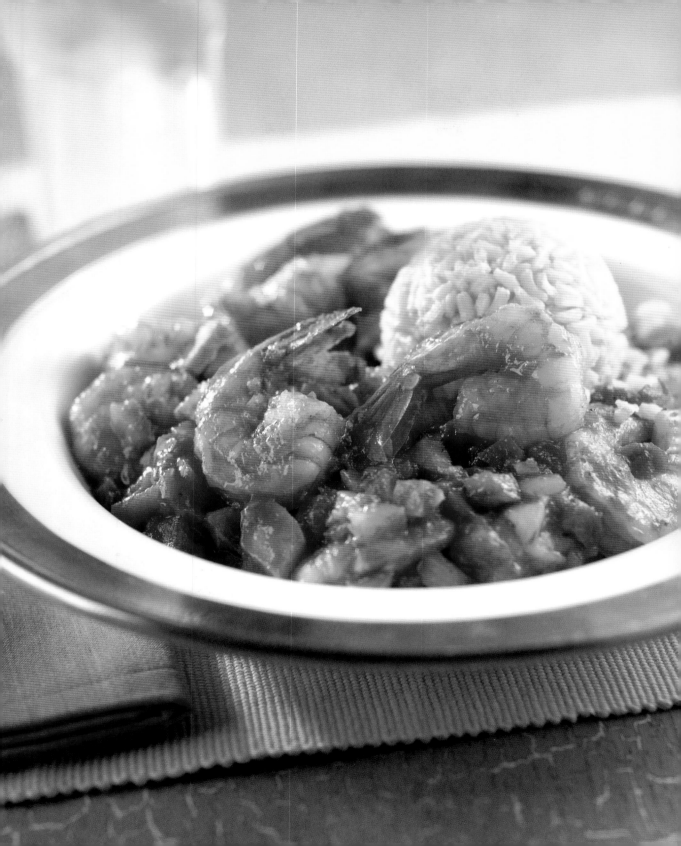

Caribbean Baked Chicken with Mango

Bake up this chicken for an authentic taste of Jamaica.

2 jalapeño chillies, halved and seeded
(wear rubber gloves when handling)

½ onion, halved

2 cloves garlic, finely chopped

1 slice (5 mm/¼ in thick) peeled fresh ginger

1 tablespoon extra virgin olive oil

1 tablespoon white wine vinegar

1 teaspoon jerk seasoning

1 teaspoon ground allspice

¼ teaspoon salt

4 boneless, skinless chicken breasts

½ mango, peeled and finely chopped

1 tablespoon chopped fresh coriander

Preheat the oven to 230°C/450°F/gas 8. Coat a small roasting tin with cooking spray.

In a food processor, combine the chillies, onion, garlic, ginger, oil, vinegar, jerk seasoning, allspice and salt. Process until very finely chopped, stopping the machine a few times to scrape down the sides of the container.

Spread the spice mixture all over the chicken breasts. Place the chicken breasts, skinned side up, in the prepared roasting tin and cook for 30 minutes, or until a thermometer inserted in the thickest part registers 75°C/170°F and the juices run clear.

Serve the chicken on warmed plates and scatter the mango and coriander on top.

Makes 4 servings

NUTRITION AT A GLANCE
Per serving: Energy 189 cals/791 kJ; 6 g fat (of which 1.5 g saturates), 27 g protein, 6 g carbohydrate (of which 5 g sugars), 1 g fibre, 283 mg sodium

Tropical Glazed Chicken

Pineapple juice and honey with a hint of mustard and cayenne pepper give this chicken a delightful sweet-and-spicy punch. You can prepare the glaze ahead, making this an easy dish for a busy evening.

240 ml (8 fl oz)	chicken stock
3	tablespoons pineapple juice
1	tablespoon coarse-grain Dijon mustard
1	clove garlic, finely chopped
1	teaspoon finely chopped fresh sage
½	teaspoon mustard powder
	dash of cayenne pepper
1	tablespoon honey
4	boneless, skinless chicken breasts

Bring the chicken stock to the boil in a small saucepan over medium-high heat until it is reduced to 4 tablespoons. Add the juice, mustard, garlic, sage, mustard powder, cayenne pepper and honey. Bring to the boil, reduce the heat to low and simmer for 5 minutes, stirring occasionally. Remove from the heat. Use immediately or store in a covered container in the refrigerator.

Coat a grill rack with cooking spray. Preheat the grill for 10 minutes on medium-high.

Grill the chicken for 4 minutes. Turn and grill the other side for 1 minute. Brush with the pineapple-mustard glaze. Grill for a further 4 minutes, brushing again with the glaze, until a thermometer inserted in the thickest part registers 75°C/170°F and the juices run clear.

Makes 4 servings

NUTRITION AT A GLANCE
Per serving: Energy 169 cals/707 kJ; 4 g fat (of which 1 g saturates), 27 g protein, 6 g carbohydrate (of which 6 g sugars), 0 g fibre, 380 mg sodium

Coconut Chicken

Chicken braised in coconut milk (Opor Ayam) *is a classic of Indonesian cuisine. We've changed the traditional drumstick or wing to the leaner white meat – new traditions can sometimes be better than old ones. Glazed Peppers and Mangetouts (see page 143) make a colourful accompaniment.*

2 tablespoons extra virgin olive oil	⅛ teaspoon ground cumin
	pinch of ground turmeric
4 boneless, skinless chicken breasts, cut into strips	240 ml (8 fl oz) coconut milk (no sugar added)
1 tablespoon chicken stock	2 tablespoons macadamia nuts, finely ground
1 onion, chopped	
2 cloves garlic, finely chopped	1 teaspoon sugar substitute
¾ teaspoon ground coriander	¼ teaspoon cayenne pepper
	1 tablespoon tamarind paste
1 teaspoon grated fresh ginger	2 teaspoons water
1 teaspoon finely grated lemon zest	chopped spring onion, to garnish

Heat the oil in a large frying pan over medium–high heat. Add the chicken and cook for 5 minutes on each side, or until browned and no longer pink in the centre. Transfer the chicken to a plate and set aside.

Add the stock to the pan, together with the onion, garlic, coriander, ginger, lemon zest, cumin and turmeric and cook for 5 minutes, or until the onion is tender but not browned. Stir in the coconut milk, nuts, sugar substitute and cayenne pepper. Return the chicken to the pan, cover and simmer for 10 minutes, or until the chicken is cooked through.

Transfer the chicken to a plate and keep warm.

In a cup, combine the tamarind paste and water. Stir into the sauce in the frying pan and simmer until thickened and the mixture measures about 240 ml (8 fl oz).

Divide the chicken among 4 serving plates. Top with sauce and garnish with the spring onion.

Makes 4 servings

NUTRITION AT A GLANCE
Per serving: Energy 285 cals/1193 kJ; 16 g fat (of which 3 g saturates), 29 g protein, 7 g carbohydrate (of which 5 g sugars), 1 g fibre, 146 mg sodium

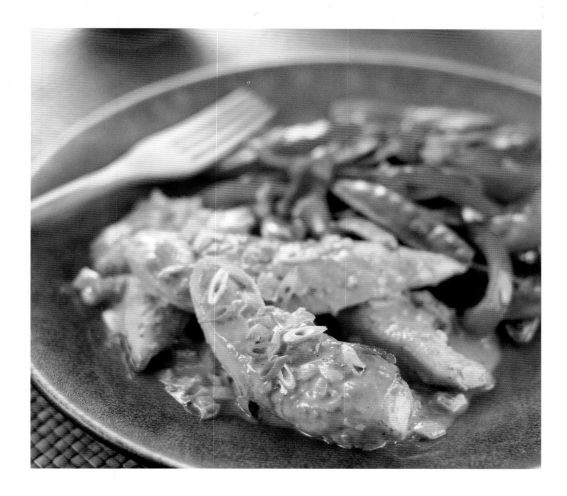

Chicken with Lime Dressing

This Tex-Mex-style chicken is sure to become a favourite. It will turn your home into a hacienda for the evening.

Lime Dressing

80 ml (3 fl oz)	fresh lime juice
4	tablespoons chopped fresh coriander
1	tablespoon finely chopped spring onions
1	tablespoon extra virgin olive oil
1	teaspoon sugar substitute
½	teaspoon salt

Mashed Avocados

2	ripe avocados, peeled and pitted
1	tablespoon fresh lemon juice
2	teaspoons salsa (not too chunky)

Chicken

4	boneless, skinless chicken breasts, pounded to 1 cm (½ in) thickness
1	teaspoon + 1 tablespoon extra virgin olive oil
1	red pepper (capsicum), finely chopped
1	clove garlic, finely chopped
30 g (1 oz)	sliced almonds, toasted
2	tablespoons wholemeal flour

To make the dressing: In a large bowl, combine the lime juice, coriander, spring onions, oil, sugar substitute and salt.

To make the mashed avocados: In a medium bowl, mash the avocados with 2 tablespoons of the lime dressing. Stir in the lemon juice and salsa.

To cook the chicken: In a large glass dish, combine the chicken with 3 tablespoons of the lime dressing. Cover and refrigerate for 10 minutes.

Heat 1 teaspoon of the oil in a large non-stick frying pan. Add the red pepper and cook, stirring occasionally, for 6 minutes, or until the pepper is tender and lightly browned. Stir in the garlic and cook for 30 seconds. Transfer to a large bowl and add the almonds.

Remove the chicken from the dressing and pat dry with paper towels. Toss the chicken in the flour.

Heat the remaining 1 tablespoon oil in the frying pan over medium-high heat. Add the chicken and cook for 6 minutes on each side, or until a thermometer inserted in the thickest part registers 75°C/170°F and the juices run clear. Place the chicken on 4 serving plates and sprinkle the pepper mixture over the chicken. Drizzle the remaining lime dressing over each serving. Serve with the mashed avocados.

Makes 4 servings

NUTRITION AT A GLANCE
Per serving: Energy 435 cals/1820 kJ; 29 g fat (of which 5 g saturates), 31 g protein, 12 g carbohydrate (of which 4 g sugars), 5 g fibre, 387 mg sodium

From the Menu of . . .

BOLO RESTAURANT & BAR

23 E. 22nd Street, New York City, New York

CHEF BOBBY FLAY

Bobby Flay is a great chef who takes part in the South Beach Wine and Food Festival. His restaurants in New York are always hoppin'.

Spanish Spice-Rubbed Chicken with Mustard and Spring Onion Dressing

PHASE 1

Mustard and Spring Onion Dressing

120 ml (4 fl oz)	white wine vinegar
3	tablespoons Dijon mustard
240 ml (8 fl oz)	extra virgin olive oil
	salt
	freshly ground black pepper
3	spring onions, thinly sliced
3	tablespoons finely chopped fresh flat-leaved parsley

Spanish Spice Rub

3	tablespoons paprika
1	tablespoon cumin seeds, ground
1	tablespoon mustard seeds, ground
2	teaspoons fennel seeds, ground
2	teaspoons coarsely ground black pepper
2	teaspoons sea salt

Chicken

8	bone-in chicken breasts
	sprigs of parsley, to garnish

To make the dressing: In a large bowl, whisk together the vinegar and mustard. Slowly whisk in the oil until emulsified. Season with salt and pepper to taste. Fold in the spring onions and parsley.

To make the spice rub: Place all the ingredients in a small bowl and mix well.

To cook the chicken: Heat the grill or a ridged grilling pan to medium. Brush the chicken breasts with olive oil. Season each chicken breast with salt on both sides. Rub each chicken breast on the skinned side with the spice rub and grill, with the rub-side nearest the heat. Grill for 5 to 6 minutes or until slightly charred and a crust has formed. Turn the chicken breasts over and continue cooking for 6 to 7 minutes or until just cooked through. Spoon some of the Mustard and Spring Onion Dressing onto each plate and place a chicken breast on top. Garnish with parsley and serve the remaining dressing separately.

Makes 8 servings

NUTRITION AT A GLANCE
Per serving: Energy 545 cals/2281 kJ; 45 g fat (of which 9 g saturates), 28 g protein, 2 g carbohydrate (of which 0.5 g sugars), 0 g fibre, 1028 mg sodium

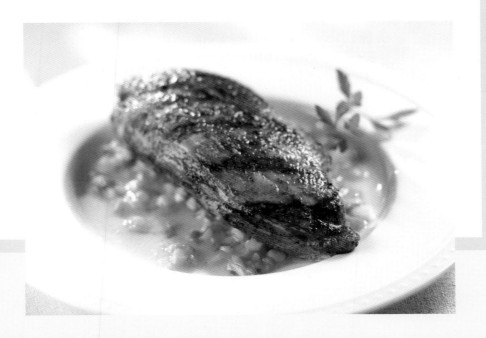

Chicken Mole

This delicious, spicy chicken will be perfect for you chocolate lovers out there.

570 g (1¼ lb)	boneless, skinless chicken breasts, cut into strips
	salt
	ground black pepper
1	large onion, chopped
1	large green pepper (capsicum), cored, seeded and chopped
2	cloves garlic, finely chopped
2	tablespoons chilli powder
½	teaspoon ground cinnamon
½	teaspoon ground cloves
400 g (14 oz)	tinned chopped tomatoes
2	tablespoons unsweetened peanut butter
2	tablespoons unsweetened cocoa powder
2	spring onions, chopped

Sprinkle the chicken with salt and black pepper. Coat a large non-stick frying pan with olive oil cooking spray and place over medium–high heat. Add the chicken and cook for 8 minutes, turning once, or until browned on both sides. Transfer the chicken to a large plate.

Add the onion, green pepper and garlic to the frying pan and cook for 3 minutes, or until the onion becomes translucent. Stir in the chilli powder, cinnamon and cloves and cook for 1 minute. Return the chicken to the pan. Add the tomatoes (with juice), peanut butter and cocoa powder and bring to the boil. Cover and simmer, stirring every few minutes, for 25 minutes, turning once, or until the chicken is no longer pink. Garnish with the spring onions.

Makes 4 servings

NUTRITION AT A GLANCE
Per serving: Energy 383 cals/1603 kJ; 18 g fat (of which 5 g saturates), 46 g protein, 12 g carbohydrate (of which 8 g sugars), 4 g fibre, 646 mg sodium

Artichoke Chicken

In the US, 16 March is National Artichoke Day. But you could serve this any day!

4	tablespoons extra virgin olive oil
4	boneless, skinless chicken breasts, pounded to 1 cm (½ in) thickness
455 g (1 lb)	fresh or frozen baby onions, peeled and blanched or thawed
400 ml (14 fl oz)	chicken stock
1	tablespoon balsamic vinegar
	salt
	ground black pepper
285 g (10 oz)	frozen artichoke hearts or artichoke hearts in olive oil, drained

Heat 2 tablespoons of the oil in a large frying pan over medium heat. Add the chicken and cook for 10 minutes, turning once, or until browned on both sides. Carefully transfer the chicken to a large plate.

Heat the remaining 2 tablespoons oil in the frying pan. Add the onions and cook, stirring occasionally, for 5 minutes, or until lightly browned. Return the chicken to the pan and add the stock and vinegar, and season with salt and pepper. Bring to the boil. Reduce the heat to low, cover and simmer for 20 minutes.

Add the artichoke hearts and cook for 10 minutes, or until the artichokes are tender and a thermometer inserted in the thickest part of a chicken breast registers 75°C/170°F and the juices run clear.

Makes 4 servings

NUTRITION AT A GLANCE
Per serving: Energy 302 cals/1264 kJ; 16 g fat (of which 3 g saturates), 30 g protein, 11 g carbohydrate (of which 8 g sugars), 3 g fibre, 466 mg sodium

Spice-Rubbed Chicken with Coriander Dipping Sauce

The vividly flavoured green dipping sauce is the perfect accompaniment, but if you prefer, you can substitute South Beach Barbecue Sauce (see page 162).

1 teaspoon chilli powder	1 clove garlic, chopped
1 teaspoon ground cumin	1 serrano (hot green) chilli, seeded (wear rubber gloves when handling)
¼ teaspoon salt	
4 boneless, skinless chicken breasts, each cut into 3 pieces	⅛ teaspoon salt
	2 tablespoons lime juice
8 tablespoons fresh coriander leaves	2 tablespoons extra virgin olive oil
4 tablespoons fresh parsley leaves	2 tablespoons water
30 g (1 oz) blanched slivered almonds	sprigs of coriander, to garnish

In a cup, combine the chilli powder, cumin and salt. Cut two 1 cm (½ in) deep slashes in each piece of chicken. Rub the spice mixture over the chicken, pressing it into the slits. Place the chicken in a dish and coat completely with cooking spray. Leave to stand for 10 minutes.

In a food processor, combine the coriander, parsley, almonds, garlic, chilli and salt. Process until chopped. While the machine is running, add the lime juice and oil through the feed tube, stopping the machine once or twice to scrape down the sides of the container, until the sauce is smooth. Pour the sauce into a bowl. Stir in the water, cover and chill until ready to serve.

Coat a grill rack with cooking spray. Preheat the grill.

Place the chicken on the prepared rack and grill 15 cm (6 in) from the heat, turning several times, for 15 minutes, or until a thermometer inserted in the thickest part registers 75°C/170°F and the juices run clear. Serve with the sauce and garnish with the coriander.

Makes 4 servings

NUTRITION AT A GLANCE
Per serving: Energy 241 cals/1008 kJ; 14 g fat (of which 2 g saturates), 28 g protein, 2 g carbohydrate (of which 1 g sugars), 1 g fibre, 492 mg sodium

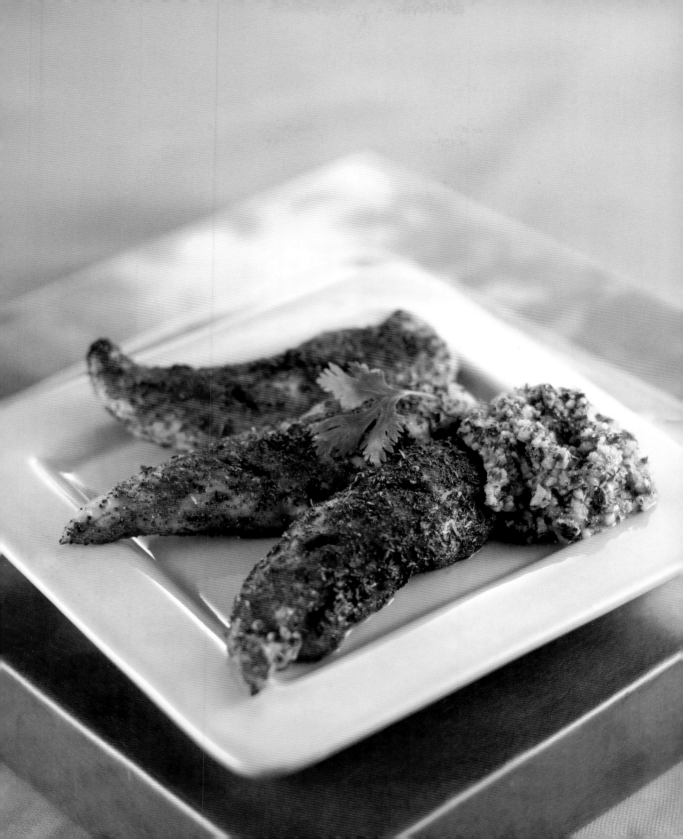

Chicken Capri

This dish tastes like it took you all day, but it can be made in 45 minutes. It goes especially well with a crisp garden salad topped with any South Beach-approved dressing.

250 g (9 oz)	ricotta cheese (reduced-fat if available)
½	teaspoon dried oregano
¼	teaspoon salt
¼	teaspoon ground black pepper
4	boneless, skinless chicken breasts
½	teaspoon garlic powder
2	tablespoons extra virgin olive oil
170 g (6 oz)	ripe, well-flavoured tomatoes, chopped
4	slices reduced-fat mozzarella cheese

In a small bowl, combine the ricotta with the oregano, salt and pepper until blended.

Rub the chicken with the garlic powder. Heat the oil in a large frying pan over medium–high heat. Add the chicken and cook for 12 minutes on each side. Place the chicken breasts side by side in a baking dish and leave to cool.

Preheat the oven to 180°C/350°F/gas 4.

Spoon a quarter of the cheese mixture and a quarter of the tomatoes onto each chicken breast. Top each chicken breast with a slice of mozzarella and cook for 20 minutes, or until a thermometer inserted in the thickest part of a breast registers 75°C/170°F and the juices run clear.

Makes 4 servings

NUTRITION AT A GLANCE
Per serving: Energy 334 cals/1398 kJ; 20 g fat (of which 9 g saturates), 34 g protein, 4 g carbohydrate (of which 3 g sugars), 0.5 g fibre, 429 mg sodium

Spicy Chinese Chicken Kebabs

These sensational skewers are excellent served hot or chilled. Serve them with hot brown rice and a salad of mixed lettuce leaves to round out the meal.

2	tablespoons orange juice
1½	tablespoons hoisin sauce
1	tablespoon South Beach Ketchup (see page 163) or sugar-free ketchup
1	tablespoon rice vinegar
1	tablespoon Chinese chilli sauce with garlic
1	teaspoon light soy sauce
1	teaspoon toasted sesame oil
1	teaspoon grated orange zest
685 g (1½ lb)	boneless, skinless chicken breasts, cut into 2.5 cm (1 in) pieces

In a large, sealable plastic bag, combine the orange juice, hoisin sauce, ketchup, vinegar, chilli sauce, soy sauce, oil and orange zest. Add the chicken. Seal the bag securely and turn to coat the chicken. Refrigerate the chicken for at least 2 hours, turning the bag occasionally.

Coat a grill rack or ridged grilling pan with cooking spray. Preheat the grill or pan.

Thread the chicken pieces onto 6 metal skewers. Grill for 5 to 7 minutes on each side, or until a thermometer inserted in the thickest part registers 75°C/170°F and the juices run clear.

Makes 6 servings

NUTRITION AT A GLANCE
Per serving: Energy 148 cals/619 kJ; 4 g fat (of which 1 g saturates), 26 g protein, 2 g carbohydrate (of which 1.5 g sugars), 0 g fibre, 455 mg sodium

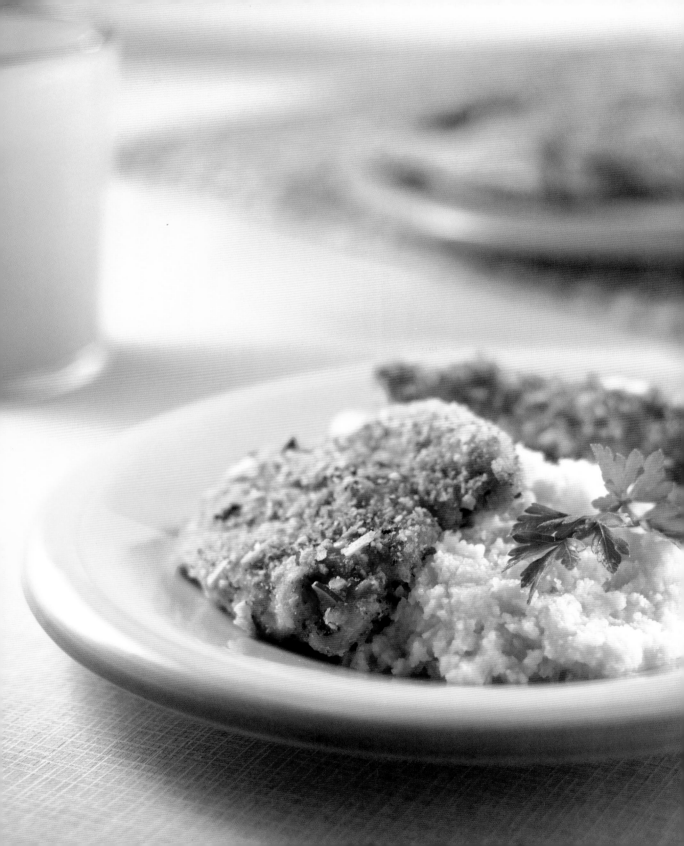

Oven-Fried Chicken with Almonds

All the delicious flavour of spicy fried chicken – with a fraction of the fat. Serve with South Beach 'Mashed Potatoes' (see page 154).

4	slices day-old wholemeal bread, crusts removed
30 g (1 oz)	Parmesan cheese, grated
30 g (1 oz)	almonds, finely chopped
2	tablespoons chopped fresh parsley
1	clove garlic, crushed
1	teaspoon salt
¼	teaspoon dried thyme
	pinch of ground black pepper
4	tablespoons extra virgin olive oil
900 g (2 lb)	boneless, skinless chicken breasts, pounded to 1 cm (½ in) thickness and cut into 12 pieces
	sprigs of flat-leaved parsley, to garnish

Preheat the oven to 110°C/250°F/gas ½. Place the bread on a baking sheet in the oven for 20 to 30 minutes, or until dry. Leave to cool. Place in a food processor and blend to fine crumbs.

Increase the oven temperature to 200°C/400°F/gas 6.

In a medium bowl, combine the breadcrumbs, cheese, almonds, parsley, garlic, salt, thyme and pepper. Mix thoroughly.

Place the oil in a shallow dish. Dip the chicken in the oil, then dredge in the crumb mixture. Place the chicken in a shallow baking tin and cook for 25 minutes, or until a thermometer inserted in the centre of a piece registers 75°C/170°F and the juices run clear. (Do not turn the chicken during cooking.) Garnish with the parsley.

Makes 6 servings

NUTRITION AT A GLANCE
Per serving: Energy 331 cals/1385 kJ; 17 g fat (of which 4 g saturates), 37 g protein, 8 g carbohydrate (of which 0.5 g sugars), 1.5 g fibre, 645 mg sodium

Five-Spice Chicken

Ginger, soy sauce and Chinese five-spice powder combine to give this spicy dinner its eastern flair.

- 3 tablespoons dry sherry
- 2 tablespoons light soy sauce
- 1 tablespoon sugar substitute (use brown sugar substitute or brown sugar substitute syrup if available)
- 1 teaspoon finely chopped fresh ginger
- 1 clove garlic, finely chopped
- ½ teaspoon Chinese five-spice powder
- 4 boneless, skinless chicken breasts
- 1 teaspoon cornflour
- 1 tablespoon cold water
- 2 spring onions, thinly sliced, to garnish

In a shallow 1.5–litre (2½–pint) microwaveable dish, combine the sherry, soy sauce, sugar substitute, ginger, garlic and five-spice powder. Add the chicken and turn to coat. Cover with vented plastic wrap and microwave for 5 minutes on high power. Turn the chicken and cook for a further 5 minutes, or until a thermometer inserted in the thickest part of a breast registers 75°C/170°F and the juices run clear. Transfer the chicken to a serving platter.

In a cup, dissolve the cornflour in the water and stir into the chicken juices. Cover with vented plastic wrap and microwave on high power for 1½ minutes. Stir and pour over the chicken. Sprinkle the spring onions over the top.

Makes 4 servings

NUTRITION AT A GLANCE
Per serving: Energy 164 cals/686 kJ; 4 g fat (of which 1 g saturates), 27 g protein, 3 g carbohydrate (of which 0.5 g sugars), 0 g fibre, 518 mg sodium

Ginger Chicken

The slightly hot taste and wonderful aroma of the ginger adds great depth of flavour to the teriyaki sauce.

1	piece (15 cm/6 in) fresh ginger, peeled and cut into 2 cm (¾ in) pieces
2	cloves garlic
2	tablespoons extra virgin olive oil
120 ml (4 fl oz)	South Beach Teriyaki Sauce (see page 163)
4	boneless, skinless chicken breasts
	salt
	ground black pepper

Preheat the oven to 230°C/450°F/gas 8.

In a blender or food processor, combine the ginger, garlic and oil. Process until finely chopped. While the machine is running, add the teriyaki sauce until the mixture has a mustard-like texture.

Place the chicken in a large, shallow bowl and cover it with the ginger mixture. Cover and refrigerate for 10 minutes.

Place the chicken on a rack in a roasting tin, season with salt and pepper and cook for about 15 minutes. Reduce the oven temperature to 180°C/350°F/gas 4. Cook the chicken for a further 5 to 10 minutes, or until a thermometer inserted in the thickest portion registers 75°C/170°F and the juices run clear.

Makes 4 servings

NUTRITION AT A GLANCE
Per serving: Energy 250 cals/1046 kJ; 11 g fat (of which 2 g saturates), 27 g protein, 6 g carbohydrate (of which 0.5 g sugars), 0 g fibre, 645 mg sodium

DORAKU

1104 Lincoln Road, Miami Beach, Florida

CHEF HIROYUKI 'HIRO' TERADA

Doraku means 'Joy of' in Japanese, and at this sushi-and-sake restaurant there's plenty to be happy about. The menu also features a selection of Asian grilled dishes.

Japanese Baked Poussin

PHASE 1

4	tablespoons light soy sauce	1	poussin (small chicken), weighing about 455 g (1 lb)
4	tablespoons water	2	teaspoons sesame oil
2	cloves garlic, finely chopped	3	asparagus spears
1	tablespoon chopped fresh ginger		

In a large bowl, mix the soy sauce, water, garlic and ginger. Place the poussin in the mixture and leave to marinate for 1 hour.

Remove the poussin from the marinade and pat dry with paper towels.

Preheat a sauté pan or grill pan and preheat the oven to 200°C/400°F/gas 6.

In the sauté pan, brown the poussin on all sides over medium–high heat. Place the poussin in a baking dish. Cut through the skin along the breastbone of the poussin.

Spoon the sesame oil over the poussin and cook for 15 to 20 minutes, or until a thermometer inserted in the thickest portion registers 75°C/170°F and the juices run clear.

Remove and discard the skin from the poussin.

Steam the asparagus for 1½ minutes, until crisp-tender.

Serve the poussin with the asparagus, pouring the pan juices over the poussin and asparagus.

Makes 1 serving

NUTRITION AT A GLANCE

Per serving: Energy 450 cals/1883 kJ; 18 g fat (of which 5 g saturates), 60 g protein, 8 g carbohydrate (of which 1 g sugars), 1.5 g fibre, 3000 mg sodium

Sesame Baked Chicken

The mild, nutty flavour of sesame seeds and sesame oil lifts this chicken dish out of the everyday.

1	egg, lightly beaten
2	tablespoons rapeseed (canola) oil
1	teaspoon toasted sesame oil
1	tablespoon water
1	tablespoon light soy sauce
½	teaspoon salt
¼	teaspoon ground black pepper
2	tablespoons oat bran
4	tablespoons sesame seeds
685 g (1½ lb)	boneless, skinless chicken breasts, cut into 5 cm (2 in) pieces

Preheat the oven to 180°C/350°F/gas 4.

In a shallow bowl, combine the egg, rapeseed oil, sesame oil, water, soy sauce, salt and pepper.

In a small bowl, combine the oat bran and sesame seeds.

Dip the chicken in the egg mixture, then dredge in the bran mixture. Place the chicken in a small non-stick roasting tin and cook for 30 minutes, or until a thermometer inserted in the centre of a piece registers 75°C/170°F and the juices run clear.

Makes 4 servings

NUTRITION AT A GLANCE
Per serving: Energy 363 cals/1519 kJ; 20 g fat (of which 3 g saturates), 43 g protein, 2.5 g carbohydrate (of which 0.5 g sugars), 4 g fibre, 651 mg sodium

Grilled Raspberry Chicken

A delicious taste of summer, to make the most of fresh raspberries, although you can also use frozen berries.

120 ml (4 fl oz)	raspberry vinegar
120 ml (4 fl oz)	red wine
60 ml (2 fl oz)	Worcestershire sauce
4	cloves garlic, finely chopped
1	teaspoon black pepper
	boneless, skinless chicken breasts
750 g (1 lb 10 oz)	cooked brown and wild rice pilaf
	sprigs of watercress or parsley, to garnish
	fresh or frozen raspberries, to garnish (thawed, if frozen)

In a large glass dish, combine the vinegar, wine, Worcestershire sauce, garlic and pepper. Place the chicken in the dish, turning to coat both sides. Cover and refrigerate for 1 hour, turning the chicken after 30 minutes.

Coat a grill rack or ridged grilling pan with cooking spray. Preheat the grill or pan.

Grill the chicken over medium-high heat, turning halfway through and brushing frequently with the marinade, for 15 minutes, or until a thermometer inserted in the thickest part registers 75°C/170°F and the juices run clear.

Arrange the chicken on the hot pilaf on a serving platter and garnish with the watercress or parsley and raspberries.

Makes 8 servings

NUTRITION AT A GLANCE
Per serving: Energy 282 cals/1180 kJ; 5 g fat (of which 1 g saturates), 28 g protein, 31 g carbohydrate (of which 1 g sugars), 1 g fibre, 516 mg sodium

Chicken and Aubergine Casserole

Chicken mixed with hearty vegetables and a hint of cheese makes a glorious combination in this casserole. Make this dish ahead and cook it the next day, or make two batches and freeze one for an easy meal another day.

1	aubergine (eggplant), peeled and cut into 12 slices
2	tablespoons grated Parmesan cheese
½	teaspoon garlic powder or 1 clove garlic, finely chopped
340 g (12 oz)	boneless, skinless chicken breast, chopped
400 g (14 oz)	tinned chopped tomatoes
1	medium onion, chopped
1	large green pepper (capsicum), chopped
90 g (3 oz)	mushrooms, sliced
¾	teaspoon dried Italian herb seasoning
¼	teaspoon ground black pepper
30 g (1 oz)	reduced-fat mozzarella cheese, grated

Preheat the grill.

Arrange the aubergine slices in a single layer on a non-stick baking sheet. Mist the slices with cooking spray. Grill 10 cm (4 in) from the heat for 2 minutes, or until golden. Turn the aubergine over and spray again. Sprinkle with the Parmesan cheese and garlic. Grill for a further 1 minute, or until golden. Set aside.

Coat a non-stick frying pan with cooking spray and place over medium–high heat for 1 minute. Add the chicken and cook, stirring often, for 5 minutes, or until no longer pink. Add the tomatoes (with juice), onion, pepper, mushrooms, herb seasoning and black pepper, stirring to break up the tomatoes. Bring to the boil. Reduce the heat to low and simmer for 5 minutes.

Preheat the oven to 190°C/375°F/gas 5.

Coat a 20 cm (8 in) square baking dish with cooking spray. Arrange 6 aubergine slices in the bottom of the dish. Top with the chicken mixture. Arrange the remaining 6 aubergine slices over the chicken. Sprinkle with the mozzarella cheese. Cover with foil and finish cooking, or refrigerate until the next day. Or wrap with foil, label, and freeze for up to 3 weeks.

Bake, covered, for 30 minutes, or until heated through.

To cook from frozen, bake, covered, at 190°C/375°F/gas 5 for 50 minutes, or until heated through.

Makes 4 servings

NUTRITION AT A GLANCE
Per serving: Energy 200 cals/837 kJ; 6 g fat (of which 3 g saturates), 26 g protein, 8 g carbohydrate (of which 6 g sugars), 3 g fibre, 237 mg sodium

Spinach-Stuffed Chicken

This tasty chicken is packed with flavour.

150 g (5 oz) frozen chopped spinach, thawed and squeezed dry

1 spring onion, chopped

3 tablespoons grated Parmesan cheese

salt

freshly ground pepper

2 thick rashers of lean back bacon, cut into strips 5 mm (¼ in) wide

4 boneless, skinless chicken breasts

1 tablespoon extra virgin olive oil

2 tablespoons white wine vinegar

4 teaspoons unsalted butter

1 tablespoon chopped fresh parsley

lemon slices, to garnish

sprigs of parsley, to garnish

Preheat the oven to 180°C/350°F/gas 4.

In a bowl, combine the spinach, spring onion and Parmesan; season to taste with salt and pepper. In a large, non-stick frying pan, cook the bacon over medium–high heat until crisp, about 4 minutes. Add the bacon to the spinach and mix well, reserving any bacon fat in the pan.

Using a sharp knife, cut a horizontal slit in each chicken breast to make a pocket. Season the chicken with salt and pepper. Spoon the spinach mixture into the chicken pockets. Add the olive oil to the frying pan and heat until sizzling. Add the chicken and cook over medium–high heat, turning once, until well browned, about 6 minutes.

Transfer the chicken breasts to an ovenproof dish. Cook in the oven for 30 minutes, or until a thermometer inserted in the thickest part registers 75°C/170°F and the juices run clear.

Transfer the chicken to 4 warmed plates. Add the vinegar to the frying pan and cook for 30 seconds. Remove the pan from the heat, add the butter and swirl until melted. Spoon the sauce over the chicken and sprinkle with chopped parsley. Garnish with lemon slices and parsley sprigs.

Makes 4 servings

NUTRITION AT A GLANCE
Per serving: Energy 275 cals/1151 kJ; 15 g fat (of which 6 g saturates), 34 g protein, 1 g carbohydrate (of which 0.5 g sugars), 1 g fibre, 635 mg sodium

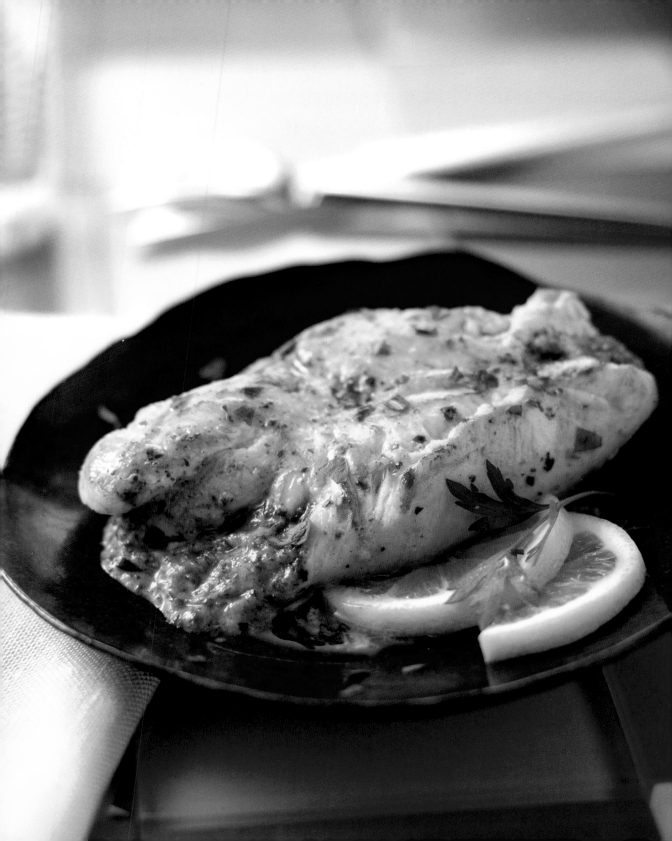

Creamy Chicken Paprikash

Inspired by a traditional Hungarian dish, this is a simple, healthy version of the original. If you want to use regular pasta, you can substitute it once in a while for the wholewheat for a Phase 3 dinner.

230 g (8 oz)	wholewheat tagliatelle, linguine or spaghetti
4	boneless, skinless chicken breasts, cut into bite-size pieces
½	teaspoon salt
¼	teaspoon ground black pepper
1	large onion, chopped
1	clove garlic, finely chopped
180 ml (6 fl oz)	chicken stock
2	teaspoons paprika
115 g (4 oz)	broccoli florets
230 g (8 oz)	fat-free natural yogurt

Sprinkle the chicken with the salt and black pepper.

Coat a large non-stick frying pan with cooking spray and place over medium heat. Add the chicken and cook, stirring, for 7 to 8 minutes, or until the pieces begin to brown. Transfer to a plate and set aside.

Add the onion, garlic and 3 tablespoons of the stock to the pan. Cook, stirring, for 5 minutes, or until the onion is tender. (Add more stock if necessary to prevent sticking.)

Stir in the paprika and cook for 1 minute. Stir in the remaining stock, then add the chicken and broccoli. Bring to the boil. Reduce the heat, cover and simmer for 20 minutes, or until the broccoli is tender.

Meanwhile, cook the pasta according to the package directions.

Stir the yogurt into the chicken mixture over low heat for 1 to 2 minutes, or until heated through; do not boil. Serve the chicken on the pasta.

Makes 4 servings

NUTRITION AT A GLANCE

Per serving: Energy 390 cals/1632 kJ; 7 g fat (of which 2 g saturates), 39 g protein, 46 g carbohydrate (of which 8 g sugars), 6 g fibre, 679 mg sodium

Wild Rice Turkey Burgers

Almost everyone likes a good burger. If only they weren't so bad for you! This recipe is the answer to the dilemma.

170 g (6 oz)	wild rice
455 g (1 lb)	turkey breast, minced
2	tablespoons South Beach Barbecue Sauce (see page 162)
1	egg, beaten
4	cubes (2.5 cm/1 in each) reduced-fat Cheddar cheese

Preheat the oven to 180°C/350°F/gas 4.

Cook the wild rice according to the package directions. Drain well.

In a large bowl, combine the turkey, wild rice, barbecue sauce and egg. Divide the turkey mixture into 4 equal parts and shape into patties, placing a cube of cheese in the centre of each patty.

Heat a large non-stick frying pan over medium–high heat. Add the patties and sear both sides. Place the patties in a non-stick baking tin and place in the oven for 10 minutes, or until a thermometer inserted in the centre of a patty registers 75°C/165°F and the meat is no longer pink.

Makes 4 servings

NUTRITION AT A GLANCE
Per serving: Energy 350 cals/1465 kJ; 7 g fat (of which 3 g saturates), 37 g protein, 35 g carbohydrate (of which 1 g sugars), 1 g fibre, 262 mg sodium

MY SOUTH BEACH DIET

IT WAS SO ENERGIZING TO SEE THE WEIGHT COMING OFF.

I started the South Beach Diet just before Thanksgiving. It was a challenge beginning just before the winter holiday season, but I was at the point of having to either go on a diet or buy all new clothes. When I heard about the South Beach Diet, I decided to give it a try. I had no idea it would become a life plan.

I'm a sunshine, sunlight person. So for me the winter can be depressing. But after starting South Beach, I had my best winter ever. It was so energizing to see the weight coming off. After losing the first 4 kg (9 lb) in just two weeks, I went on to lose a total of 11.5 kg (25 lb). At my top weight, I was 72.5 kg (11½ st); now I'm 61 kg (9½ st) – a comfortable size 12.

I won't say that Phase 1 was easy, because I love carbs . . . I really missed rice, bread and pasta. But I was encouraged by losing 4 kg (9 lb) right away, so that made it easier to stay away from them.

My mother had a stroke at the age of 60, and my dad had heart problems, so at 54, I'm pleased to be taking preventive health measures. At my last check-up, my blood pressure and cholesterol levels were excellent. I've also been walking three times a week, which helps me stay healthy and energized.

For breakfast, my husband and I love our omelettes – a favourite is with onions, asparagus and a little cheese. Lunch is easy: packaged green salads with some leftover protein from dinner, maybe some salmon or chicken that we've grilled the night before. My favourite snack is a Granny Smith apple with a little bit of peanut butter.

One of my favourite dinners is to top a small amount of wholewheat pasta with some low-fat turkey sausage, diced tomato, and spinach and bake it. It's great! The ricotta cheese dessert is wonderful, and sometimes we have a little sugar-free ice cream. For an extra treat, I'll shave a little dark chocolate on top of these desserts.

What I love is that you don't have to give up eating out on this plan; just learn to modify your food choices. My husband loves to try out fine restaurants. Even in Italian restaurants, I just order double vegetables instead of pasta, and I stay right on track.

It's great that I don't have those 'sugar lows' any more; my energy level is more even. It's easy to enjoy being on this plan. – *SHARON L.*

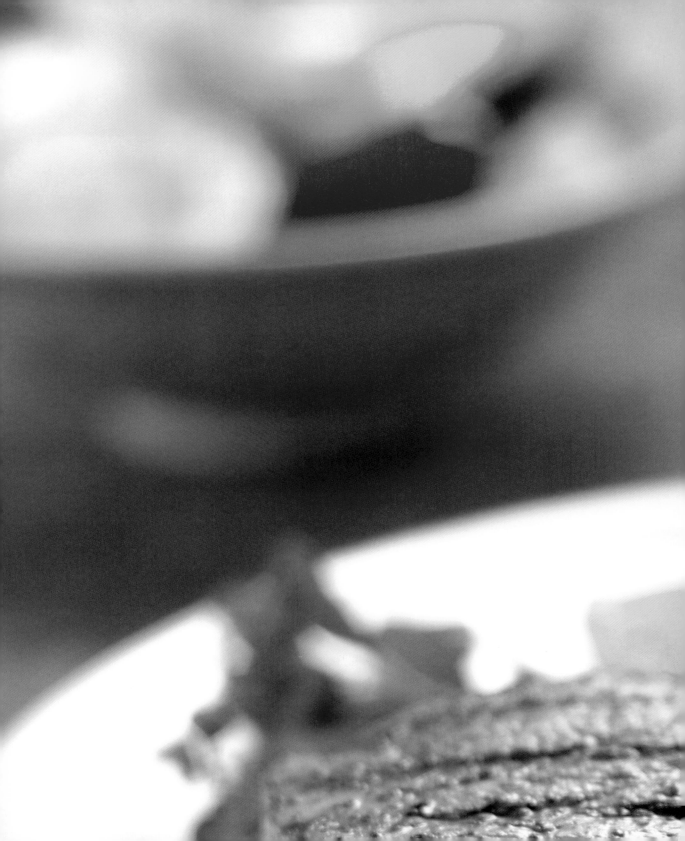

MEAT

HERE IS WHERE THE SOUTH BEACH DIET LEAST RESEMBLES A WEIGHT LOSS PROGRAMME. IN THIS CHAPTER, YOU'LL FIND QUITE A FEW RED–MEAT RECIPES, SIMPLY BECAUSE EATING BEEF NEED NOT BE UNHEALTHY OR FATTENING, DESPITE WHAT WE'VE ALL BEEN LED TO BELIEVE. THIS IS ESPECIALLY TRUE IF YOU STICK WITH THE LEANEST CUTS — FILLET STEAK, SIRLOIN (TRIMMED OF VISIBLE FAT), OR TOPSIDE. THE SATURATED FAT CONTENT OF LEAN BEEF ISN'T TERRIBLY HIGH. AND BEEF CONTAINS THE IMPORTANT NUTRIENTS IRON AND ZINC. BEST OF ALL, STEAK TASTES GOOD, AND IT WILL SATISFY YOUR HUNGER FAR BETTER THAN A BIG PLATE OF PASTA. BE SURE TO STEER CLEAR OF THE FATTIEST CUTS, INCLUDING THOSE WHERE THE MEAT IS MARBLED WITH FAT.

AND IF YOU ENJOY LAMB OR PORK, FEEL FREE TO CONTINUE DOING SO, CHOOSING LEAN CUTS AND USING THE RECIPES IN THIS CHAPTER, OR PREPARING THEM IN SIMPLE, HEALTHY WAYS — GRILLING, ROASTING, OR SAUTÉING IN EXTRA VIRGIN OLIVE OIL RATHER THAN IN BUTTER.

Beef Kebabs with Peanut Dipping Sauce

Taking their inspiration from the satay of Indonesia and Malaysia, these kebabs are naturally healthy and quick to make.

120 ml (4 fl oz) light soy sauce	1 tablespoon finely chopped fresh ginger
2 tablespoons sugar substitute (brown if available)	¼ teaspoon cayenne pepper
4 cloves garlic, crushed	1 green pepper (capsicum), cut into squares
685 g (1½ lb) sirloin steak, 4 cm (1½ in) thick, cut into 2.5 cm (1 in) pieces	1 red pepper (capsicum), cut into squares
115 g (4 oz) smooth unsweetened peanut butter	1 large onion, cut into wedges
150 ml (5 fl oz) water	
3 tablespoons lime juice	

In a shallow dish, combine half of the soy sauce, 1 tablespoon of the sugar substitute and 2 of the crushed garlic cloves. Add the steak and stir to coat. Leave to stand for 20 minutes, stirring once.

Meanwhile, in a heavy saucepan over high heat, combine the peanut butter, water, lime juice, ginger, cayenne pepper and the remaining soy sauce, sugar substitute and garlic. Cook, stirring constantly, until the mixture comes to the boil. Remove the pan from the heat.

Coat a grill rack with cooking spray. Preheat the grill to high.

Thread the steak, peppers and onion wedges onto 4 metal skewers. Grill, turning occasionally, for 10 minutes, or until the steak is cooked to your liking and the peppers and onion are beginning to brown. Serve with the peanut sauce.

Makes 4 servings

NUTRITION AT A GLANCE

Per serving: Energy 440 cals/1842 kJ; 24 g fat (of which 7 g saturates), 44 g protein, 13 g carbohydrate (of which 8 g sugars), 4 g fibre, 1068 mg sodium

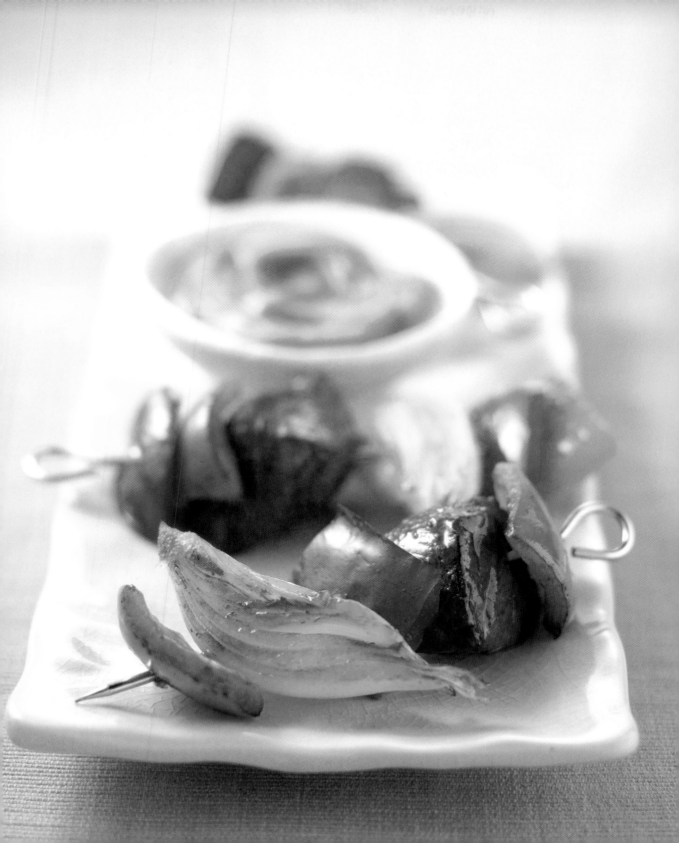

Steak and Mushroom Kebabs

Make these tasty kebabs today, and they'll be perfect for supper or a barbecue tomorrow.

120 ml (4 fl oz)	red wine
4	tablespoons extra virgin olive oil
2	tablespoons South Beach Ketchup (see page 163)
1	tablespoon vinegar
1	teaspoon Worcestershire sauce
1	clove garlic, crushed
1	teaspoon salt
½	teaspoon dried marjoram
½	teaspoon dried oregano
900 g (2 lb)	sirloin steak, cut into 5 cm (2 in) pieces
200 g (7 oz)	large button mushrooms

In a large bowl, combine the wine, oil, ketchup, vinegar, Worcestershire sauce, garlic, salt, marjoram and oregano. Add the steak and the mushrooms and stir to coat. Cover and leave to stand at room temperature for 20 minutes, then refrigerate overnight.

Coat a grill rack with cooking spray. Preheat the grill or barbecue.

Discard the marinade. Thread the meat and the mushrooms onto 4 metal skewers.

Cook over hot coals or under the grill, 10 cm (4 in) from the heat, turning occasionally, for 7 minutes, or until the meat is no longer pink.

Makes 4 servings

NUTRITION AT A GLANCE

Per serving: Energy 319 cals/1335 kJ; 13 g fat (of which 3 g saturates), 47 g protein, 0.5 g carbohydrate (of which 0 g sugars), 0.5 g fibre, 344 mg sodium

Beef Fondue

If you have time, try making an assortment of the South Beach sauces in this book, then serving them as accompaniments to this fondue of beef fillet.

900 g (2 lb) beef fillet, cut into 2.5 cm (1 in) cubes

1 recipe South Beach Teriyaki Sauce (see page 163)

1 recipe South Beach Tomato Sauce (see page 156)

1 recipe South Beach Barbecue Sauce (see page 162)

1 recipe South Beach Cocktail Sauce (see page 162)

1 recipe South Beach Ketchup (see page 163)

rapeseed (canola) oil or beef or chicken stock

Divide the beef among 4 individual dishes. Place the sauces in individual bowls. Heat the oil or stock in a fondue pot to about 190°C/375°F. Using fondue forks or skewers, dip the cubes of beef into the hot oil to cook it. Then dip the beef into one of the sauces.

Makes 4 servings

NUTRITION AT A GLANCE

Per serving: Energy 310 cals/1298 kJ; 10 g fat (of which 4 g saturates), 46 g protein, 1 g carbohydrate (of which 0.5 g sugars), 0 g fibre, 300 mg sodium

THE BILTMORE HOTEL

1200 Anastasia Avenue, Coral Gables, Florida

EXECUTIVE CHEF GEOFFREY COUSINEAU

THE OPULENT *BILTMORE HOTEL* IN CORAL GABLES, WITH ITS DISTINCTIVE GIRALDA TOWER, IS A NATIONAL HISTORIC LANDMARK.

Grilled Lamb Loin Salad
with Chilled Greek Olive Ratatouille

PHASE 1

Lamb

685 g (1½ lb)	boned lamb loin, trimmed of all visible fat
1	teaspoon extra virgin olive oil
2	tablespoons harissa paste
	sea salt
	freshly ground black pepper

Ratatouille

1	courgette (zucchini), chopped
1	yellow courgette (zucchini), chopped
1	red pepper (capsicum), chopped
1	yellow pepper (capsicum), chopped
1	small aubergine (eggplant), chopped
½	fennel bulb, chopped
60 g (2 oz)	garlic, chopped

1	teaspoon extra virgin olive oil
1	tablespoon tomato purée (concentrate)
1	teaspoon chopped fresh rosemary
1	teaspoon chopped fresh basil
1	teaspoon chopped fresh oregano
4	tablespoons aged balsamic vinegar
	salt
	pepper
60 g (2 oz)	pitted black olives, chopped, to garnish
115 g (4 oz)	feta cheese, crumbled, to garnish
2	tablespoons basil-infused olive oil, to garnish
8	sprigs of fennel, to garnish

To prepare the lamb: Rub the lamb with the olive oil, harissa paste, salt and black pepper. Wrap with plastic wrap and refrigerate overnight.

To make the ratatouille: Sauté the courgettes, peppers, aubergine, fennel and garlic in the olive oil until soft but not overcooked. Drain off excess liquid and stir in the tomato purée. Cook for a further 1 minute. Add the rosemary, basil, oregano and 2 tablespoons of the vinegar and season lightly. Place in a glass or stainless steel bowl and refrigerate overnight.

To serve: Preheat the grill. Grill the lamb until cooked to your liking and leave to rest for 10 minutes.

Firmly press the chilled ratatouille into a small ring mould (or a nice round dollop in the centre of each plate) with a spoon, dividing it among 8 plates. Slice the lamb and arrange on top of the ratatouille. Garnish with the olives, cheese, the remaining balsamic vinegar, the basil-infused olive oil and sprigs of fennel.

Makes 8 servings

NUTRITION AT A GLANCE
Per serving: Energy 269 cals/1126 kJ; 16 g fat (of which 6 g saturates), 22 g protein, 9 g carbohydrate (of which 5 g sugars), 2 g fibre, 669 mg sodium

Fillet Steak with Tomato Topping

You can enjoy this tender cut of beef in all phases of the South Beach Diet. Here, it's served topped with juicy tomatoes marinated in a mixture of garlic, herbs and soy sauce.

2	teaspoons light soy sauce
1½	teaspoons Dijon mustard
1½	teaspoons finely chopped fresh parsley
1	clove garlic, finely chopped
2	tomatoes, finely chopped
2	teaspoons extra virgin olive oil
4	fillet steaks (170 g/6 oz each and 4 cm/1½ in thick)
¼	teaspoon salt
½	teaspoon ground black pepper

Preheat the oven to 200°C/400°F/gas 6.

In a bowl, combine the soy sauce, mustard, parsley and garlic. Gently stir in the tomatoes.

Heat the oil in a large ovenproof frying pan over high heat. Season the steaks with the salt and pepper. Place the steaks in the pan and cook on one side for 4 minutes, or until well browned. Turn and brown the second side for 30 seconds. Place the pan in the oven and cook for 12 minutes, or until a thermometer inserted in the thickest part registers 70°C/160°F for medium. Serve topped with the tomatoes.

Makes 4 servings

NUTRITION AT A GLANCE
Per serving: Energy 260 cals/1088 kJ; 12 g fat (of which 4 g saturates), 35 g protein, 2 g carbohydrate (of which 1 g sugars), 0.5 g fibre, 503 mg sodium

Marinated Steak

Put the meat in the marinade before going to work, and you can prepare your meal in 15 minutes when you get home. Serve with stir-fried vegetables.

120 ml (4 fl oz)	red wine
2	teaspoons light soy sauce
	pinch of ground black pepper
¼	teaspoon dried oregano
455 g (1 lb)	topside of beef or rump steak, trimmed of all visible fat

In a shallow dish, combine the wine, soy sauce, pepper and oregano. Add the meat and turn to coat both sides with the marinade. Cover and refrigerate for at least 6 hours or overnight, turning the meat occasionally.

When ready to cook, remove the meat from the marinade, pat dry with paper towels, and discard the marinade.

Coat a grill rack with olive oil cooking spray. Preheat the grill.

Place the meat on the prepared rack. Grill 10 cm (4 in) from the heat for 5 minutes on each side, or until a thermometer inserted in the centre of the meat registers 70°C/160°F for medium.

To serve, thinly slice the meat diagonally across the grain and place on 4 warmed plates.

Makes 4 servings

NUTRITION AT A GLANCE
Per serving: Energy 145 cals/607 kJ; 5 g fat (of which 2 g saturates), 23 g protein, 0 g carbohydrate, 0 g fibre, 113 mg sodium

Steak au Poivre

This is our South Beach version of a favourite recipe.

1 clove garlic, crushed	1 yellow pepper (capsicum), cut into strips
1½ teaspoons crushed black or mixed peppercorns	½ teaspoon salt
4 fillet steaks (115 g/4 oz each), trimmed of all visible fat	1 clove garlic, finely chopped
	80 ml (3 fl oz) beef stock
½ onion, chopped	½ teaspoon paprika
1 green pepper (capsicum), cut into strips	4 tablespoons crème fraîche or light sour cream
1 red pepper (capsicum), cut into strips	

In a small bowl, combine the crushed garlic and 1 teaspoon of the peppercorns. Press a small amount of the mixture onto each side of the steaks.

Coat a large non-stick frying pan with olive oil cooking spray and place over medium heat. Arrange the steaks in the pan so that they do not overlap. Cook the steaks, turning frequently, for 5 to 10 minutes, or until a thermometer inserted in the centre of a steak registers 70°C/160°F for medium. Transfer the steaks to a serving platter and keep warm.

Clean the frying pan, coat with cooking spray and place over medium heat. Add the onion, peppers, salt and finely chopped garlic and cook, stirring occasionally, for 5 minutes. Spoon the mixture around the steaks.

In a small bowl, combine the beef stock, paprika and the remaining ½ teaspoon peppercorns. Pour into the frying pan and cook, stirring often, over medium heat until the mixture is reduced to 4 tablespoons. Add the crème fraîche or light sour cream and cook for a further 2 minutes.

Spoon the sauce over each steak and serve immediately.

Makes 4 servings

NUTRITION AT A GLANCE
Per serving: Energy 210 cals/880 kJ; 9 g fat (of which 5 g saturates), 25 g protein, 5 g carbohydrate (of which 4 g sugars), 2 g fibre, 131 mg sodium

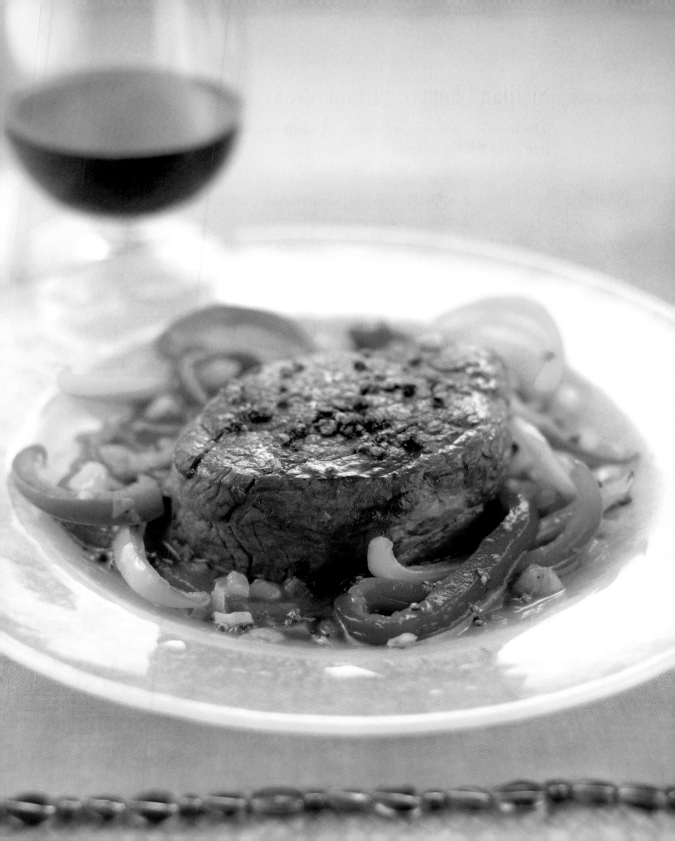

Sicilian Chopped Sirloin Steak

This lunch is a new twist on a plain old hamburger. In Phase 2 or 3, you can even add a wholemeal bun.

1	small head garlic
6	oil-packed sun-dried tomato halves, drained and finely chopped
2	tablespoons mayonnaise
685 g (1½ lb)	sirloin steak, trimmed of all visible fat, chopped
4	slices Fontina or mozzarella cheese
	rocket, to garnish
	fresh basil leaves, to garnish

Preheat the oven to 200°C/400°F/gas 6.

Wrap the garlic in foil and roast for 30 minutes, or until very tender. When cool enough to handle, squeeze the garlic pulp into a cup. Add the sun-dried tomato halves and mayonnaise. Add the steak and mix well.

Divide the steak mixture into 4 equal parts and form into patties.

Heat a large non-stick frying pan over medium heat. Add the patties and cook, turning occasionally, for 10 minutes, or until a thermometer inserted in the centre registers 70°C/160°F and the meat is no longer pink. When the patties have been turned over for the last time, place a slice of cheese on each patty. When the cheese melts, transfer the patties to 4 serving plates and garnish with the rocket and basil.

Makes 4 servings

NUTRITION AT A GLANCE

Per serving: Energy 383 cals/1603 kJ; 24 g fat (of which 7 g saturates), 39 g protein, 3 g carbohydrate (of which 2 g sugars), 1 g fibre, 233 mg sodium

Steak Diane

This simple version of the classic steak dish will appeal to everyone, regardless of diet.

4 fillet steaks (90 g/3 oz each), trimmed of all visible fat	1 small clove garlic, finely chopped
salt	1 teaspoon mustard powder
coarsely ground black pepper	1 tablespoon Worcestershire sauce
5 tablespoons trans-fat-free butter substitute	2 tablespoons lemon juice
2 shallots, finely chopped	2 tablespoons chopped fresh parsley
30 g (1 oz) mushroom caps, sliced 3 mm (⅛ in) thick	1 tablespoon chopped fresh chives

Place each steak, one at a time, between 2 pieces of greaseproof paper. Starting in the centre and working your way to the outside, pound the steaks with a meat mallet until 1 cm (½ in) thick. Dry the steaks with paper towels, then sprinkle with the salt and pepper.

In a frying pan over medium heat, melt 3 tablespoons of the butter substitute. Increase the heat to medium–high and cook each steak for 2 minutes on each side. Transfer to a plate.

In the same pan melt the remaining 2 tablespoons butter substitute. Add the shallots, mushrooms and garlic and cook, stirring, for 1 minute. Add the mustard and Worcestershire sauce and mix well. Return the steaks to the pan and cook until done to your liking. Place the steaks on warm serving plates. Add the lemon juice, parsley and chives to the pan and mix thoroughly. Cook for 30 seconds, or until just warm. Pour the sauce evenly over the steaks.

Makes 4 servings

NUTRITION AT A GLANCE
Per serving: Energy 280 cals/1172 kJ; 20 g fat (of which 5 g saturates), 20 g protein, 3 g carbohydrate (of which 1.5 g sugars), 0.5 g fibre, 652 mg sodium

Pepper-Spiked Beef Stew

Braised beef spiked with chilli pepper and other seasonings makes this stew special. It freezes well, so you might want to simmer up a double batch. You can try substituting sweet potatoes or butternut squash for the potatoes and carrots. Or, if you eliminate the potatoes, this recipe will fit into Phase 2.

2 tablespoons wholemeal flour	1 teaspoon dried oregano
1 tablespoon chilli powder	450 ml (15 fl oz) beef stock
½ teaspoon salt	2 × 400 g (14 oz) tins chopped tomatoes
900 g (2 lb) lean stewing beef, trimmed of all visible fat and cubed	½ teaspoon crushed dried chilli flakes
1 tablespoon extra virgin olive oil	1 potato, scrubbed and cubed
3 onions, sliced	4 carrots, sliced
3 cloves garlic, finely chopped	

In a large sealable plastic bag, combine the flour, 1 teaspoon of the chilli powder and the salt. Add the beef, seal the bag and toss to coat well.

Heat the oil in a large saucepan over medium–high heat. Add the beef and cook, stirring occasionally, for 7 minutes, or until browned. Add the onions, garlic and oregano. Reduce the heat to medium and cook, stirring often, for 5 minutes.

Add the stock, tomatoes (with juice), chilli flakes and the remaining 2 teaspoons chilli powder. Bring to the boil. Reduce the heat to low, cover and simmer for 2 hours, stirring occasionally, or until the beef is almost tender.

Add the potato and carrots. Cover and cook for 30 minutes, or until the vegetables are tender.

Makes 8 servings

NUTRITION AT A GLANCE

Per serving: Energy 230 cals/963 kJ; 7 g fat (of which 2 g saturates), 26 g protein, 18 g carbohydrate (of which 9 g sugars), 3 g fibre, 362 mg sodium

Roasted Aubergine Stuffed with Beef

This dish looks elaborate, but the preparation is really quite easy. You can prepare the stuffing mixture ahead and fill the aubergine (eggplant) shells just before roasting.

2 aubergines (eggplants) (455 g/1 lb each)	455 g (1 lb) extra-lean minced beef
2 tablespoons extra virgin olive oil	1½ teaspoons dried oregano
½ large onion, chopped	120 ml (4 fl oz) passata (sieved tomatoes)
1 green pepper (capsicum), chopped	60 g (2 oz) Parmesan cheese, grated
2 cloves garlic, finely chopped	¼ teaspoon salt
	¼ teaspoon ground black pepper

Preheat the oven to 200°C/400°F/gas 6.

Pierce the aubergines in 2 or 3 places and place on a baking sheet. Roast, turning once or twice, for 20 minutes, or just until tender. When cool enough to handle, halve lengthwise and scoop out the pulp, leaving a 1–2 cm (½–¾ in) shell. Set the shells aside. Chop the pulp and leave to drain in a colander.

Heat 1 tablespoon of the oil in a large frying pan over medium heat. Add the onion and pepper and cook, stirring occasionally, for 8 minutes, or until tender. Add the garlic and beef and cook, stirring to crumble the beef, for 5 minutes, or until no longer pink. Stir in the aubergine pulp, oregano and tomato passata. Reduce the heat to low and cook, stirring occasionally, for 15 minutes, or until thick. Stir in half of the cheese, the salt and black pepper.

Place the aubergine shells on a baking sheet and divide the beef mixture among them. Sprinkle with the remaining cheese and drizzle with the remaining 1 tablespoon oil. Roast for 15 minutes, or until lightly browned on top.

Makes 4 servings

NUTRITION AT A GLANCE

Per serving: Energy 298 cals/1247 kJ; 16 g fat (of which 6 g saturates), 31 g protein, 7 g carbohydrate (of which 6 g sugars), 3 g fibre, 455 mg sodium

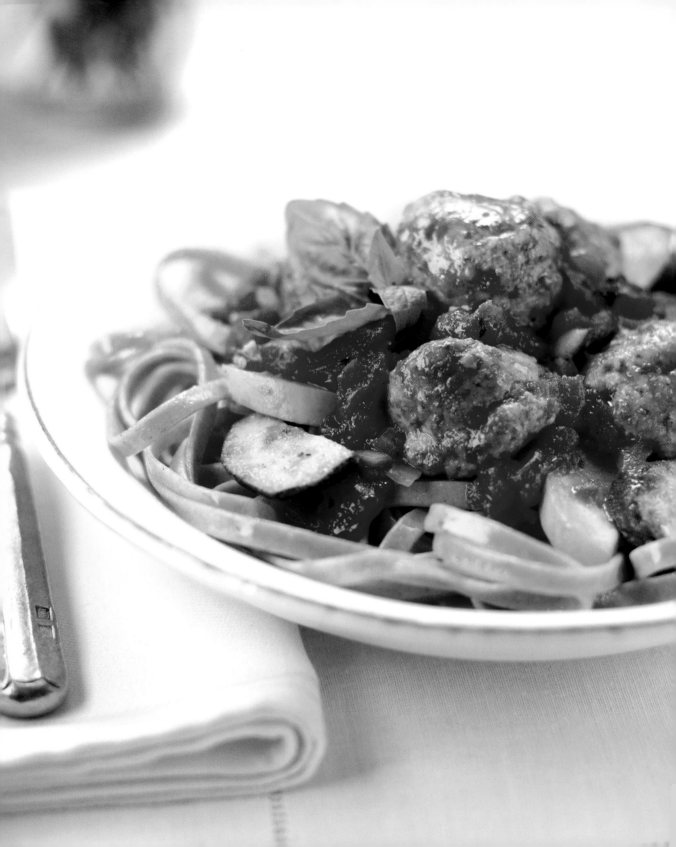

Meatballs with Tomato and Courgette Medley

Use this one-dish meal to add a few servings of vegetables to your day. Serve it in bowls with crusty multigrain bread or spoon it over wholewheat fettuccine.

230 g (8 oz) extra-lean minced beef or minced turkey breast

30 g (1 oz) fresh wholemeal breadcrumbs

1 egg

¾ teaspoon ground black pepper

½ teaspoon Italian herb seasoning

6 tablespoons grated Parmesan cheese

1 onion, finely chopped

2 cloves garlic, finely chopped

2 courgettes (zucchini), halved lengthwise and sliced

1 yellow courgette (zucchini), halved lengthwise and sliced

400 g (14 oz) tinned plum tomatoes

400 g (14 oz) tinned chopped tomatoes

4 tablespoons chopped fresh basil

sprigs of basil, to garnish

In a large bowl, combine the beef or turkey, breadcrumbs, egg, ½ teaspoon of the pepper, the Italian seasoning and 4 tablespoons of the cheese. Form into balls the size of walnuts.

Coat a large non-stick frying pan with cooking spray and place over medium–high heat. Working in batches, add the meatballs and cook for 15 minutes, or until browned and no longer pink inside. Transfer to a bowl, leaving the juices in the pan. Repeat to cook the remaining meatballs.

Add the onion and garlic to the pan and cook for 5 minutes, or until the onion is tender. Stir in the courgettes, tomatoes (with juice), the remaining ¼ teaspoon pepper, the remaining 2 tablespoons cheese and the meatballs. Bring to the boil, then reduce the heat to low, cover and cook for 20 minutes. Stir in the chopped basil. Garnish with the basil sprigs.

Makes 4 servings

NUTRITION AT A GLANCE
Per serving: Energy 261 cals/1092 kJ; 12 g fat (of which 6 g saturates), 26 g protein, 13 g carbohydrate (of which 9 g sugars), 3 g fibre, 405 mg sodium

New Beef Burgundy

This version of the familiar French boeuf bourguignonne is simple yet sophisticated. Beef, red wine, baby onions and mushrooms are the hallmarks of this dish. For a twist, there's a surprise ingredient: unsweetened cocoa powder!

30 g (1 oz)	wholemeal flour		700 ml (1¼ pints)	red wine
¼	teaspoon salt		1 litre (1¾ pints)	beef stock
¼	teaspoon ground black pepper		4	tablespoons tomato purée (concentrate)
685 g (1½ lb)	lean stewing beef, cubed		1	teaspoon unsweetened cocoa powder
2	tablespoons extra virgin olive oil		2	bay leaves
230 g (8 oz)	pearl onions		4	tablespoons chopped fresh parsley
455 g (1 lb)	button mushrooms, quartered			
3	cloves garlic, finely chopped			

In a sealable plastic bag, combine the flour, salt and pepper. Add the beef, seal the bag, and toss to coat well.

Heat 1 tablespoon of the oil in a large saucepan over medium–high heat. Working in batches to prevent overcrowding the pan, add the beef and cook, stirring frequently, for 5 minutes, or until browned. Transfer to a plate and repeat with the remaining beef.

Add the remaining 1 tablespoon oil to the pan. Add the onions, mushrooms and garlic and cook, stirring often, for 10 minutes, or until lightly browned.

Add the wine, stock, tomato purée, cocoa powder, bay leaves and beef. Bring to the boil. Reduce the heat to low, cover and simmer for 2 hours. Remove and discard the bay leaves. Sprinkle with the parsley.

Makes 8 servings

NUTRITION AT A GLANCE

Per serving: Energy 235 cals/984 kJ; 7 g fat (of which 2 g saturates), 21 g protein, 7 g carbohydrate (of which 3 g sugars), 2 g fibre, 285 mg sodium

South Beach Meat Loaf with Vegetables

Brown rice helps keeps this meat loaf moist and lends a pleasing nutty flavour that you won't find in traditional versions.

90 g (3 oz)	brown rice
1	tablespoon extra virgin olive oil
1	onion, chopped
½	red pepper (capsicum), chopped
½	green pepper (capsicum), chopped
230 g (8 oz)	extra-lean minced beef
230 g (8 oz)	minced turkey breast
250 g (9 oz)	chunky salsa
1	egg, beaten
¾	teaspoon salt
½	teaspoon ground black pepper
1	clove garlic, finely chopped

Cook the rice according to the package directions. Drain well.

Preheat the oven to 180°C/350°F/gas 4.

Heat the oil in a small frying pan over medium heat. Add the onion and peppers and cook for 5 minutes, or until tender.

In a large bowl, combine the beef, turkey, salsa, egg, salt, black pepper and garlic. Stir in the vegetables and rice. Place the mixture in a baking dish and pat into an oblong loaf.

Cook for 45 minutes, or until a thermometer inserted in the centre registers 70°C/160°F and the meat is no longer pink.

Makes 6 servings

NUTRITION AT A GLANCE
Per serving: Energy 206 cals/862 kJ; 6 g fat (of which 2 g saturates), 20 g protein, 20 g carbohydrate (of which 6 g sugars), 2 g fibre, 324 mg sodium

SMITH & WOLLENSKY

1 Washington Avenue, Miami Beach, Florida

CHEF ROBERT MIGNOLA

SMITH & WOLLENSKY IS ON THE SOUTHERN TIP OF MIAMI BEACH,
FACING FISHER ISLAND AND LOOKING OUT OVER THE BAY.
THE VIEWS ARE SPECTACULAR.

Grilled Fillet Steak with Roasted Garlic and Chipotle Pepper Chimichurri

PHASE 1

Fillet Steak

4   fillet steaks
    (170 g/6 oz each)

    salt

    freshly ground black
    pepper

Roasted Garlic and Chipotle Pepper Chimichurri

1   head garlic

1   chipotle pepper in adobo sauce

4   tablespoons extra virgin olive oil

4   tablespoons finely chopped flat-leaved parsley

    salt

    freshly ground black pepper

To make the chimichurri: Preheat the oven to 160°C/325°F/gas 3.

Cut the top 5 mm (¼ in) off the garlic to expose the cloves, wrap loosely in foil and bake for approximately 45 minutes, until the garlic is lightly browned and very soft. Leave to cool to room temperature, then squeeze out the roasted garlic.

Combine the garlic with the chipotle pepper in a food processor or blender, slowly drizzle in the oil, then stir in the parsley and season to taste with salt and pepper.

To serve: Preheat the grill. Season the steaks with salt and pepper. Grill the steaks until done to your liking, about 4 to 6 minutes on each side for medium rare. Drizzle with the chimichurri sauce.

Note: chipotle peppers (dried, smoked jalapeño chillies) are very spicy. Use more or less according to taste. Try this chimichurri sauce with grilled pork, chicken or fish.

Makes 4 servings

NUTRITION AT A GLANCE

Per serving: Energy 330 cals/1380 kJ; 20 g fat (of which 5 g saturates), 36 g protein, 4 g carbohydrate (of which 2.5 g sugars), 1 g fibre, 494 mg sodium

Pizza Meat Pie

It looks like pizza, it tastes like pizza — what's not to love about this recipe?

455 g (1 lb)	extra-lean minced beef
60 g (2 oz)	dried skimmed milk
30 g (1 oz)	fresh wholemeal breadcrumbs
1	teaspoon salt
½	teaspoon ground black pepper
1	clove garlic, crushed
115 g (4 oz)	reduced-fat mozzarella cheese, grated
2	tablespoons tomato purée (concentrate)
120 ml (4 fl oz)	water
115 g (4 oz)	mushrooms, sliced
1	teaspoon dried oregano
2	tablespoons finely chopped onion
45 g (1½ oz)	Parmesan cheese, grated

Preheat the oven to 180°C/350°F/gas 4.

In a medium bowl, combine the beef, milk, breadcrumbs, salt, pepper and garlic. Mix well. Pat the mixture into a 23 cm (9 in) pie plate.

In the same bowl, combine the mozzarella cheese, tomato purée, water, mushrooms, oregano and onion. Spoon the mixture over the meat mixture. Sprinkle with the Parmesan cheese and cook for 35 to 40 minutes, or until the meat is no longer pink.

Makes 4 servings

NUTRITION AT A GLANCE
Per serving: Energy 308 cals/1289 kJ; 11 g fat (of which 6 g saturates), 37 g protein, 15 g carbohydrate (of which 12 g sugars), 1 g fibre, 1000 mg sodium

Mexican Lasagne

Try this lasagne when you're in the mood for Mexican.

455 g (1 lb)	extra-lean minced beef or minced turkey breast	8	tablespoons chopped fresh coriander (optional)
½	large onion, chopped	2	teaspoons ground cumin
1	large clove garlic, finely chopped	⅛	teaspoon salt
230 g (8 oz)	low-fat cottage cheese or fromage frais	625 g (1 lb 6 oz)	salsa
230 g (8 oz)	fat-free natural yogurt	4	wholewheat tortillas (15 cm/6 in in diameter), halved
115 g (4 oz)	bottled chopped green chillies	115 g (4 oz)	reduced-fat Cheddar cheese, grated

Preheat the oven to 180°C/350°F/gas 4.

Coat a 32 × 23 cm (13 × 9 in) baking dish with cooking spray.

Coat a large non-stick frying pan with cooking spray and place over medium heat. Add the minced beef or turkey and cook, stirring frequently, for 5 minutes or until no longer pink.

Transfer the beef or turkey to a bowl. Wipe the pan with a paper towel. Coat the pan with cooking spray and place over medium heat. Add the onions and garlic, cover and cook, stirring occasionally, for 7 to 8 minutes, or until lightly browned. Add to the beef or turkey in the bowl.

In another bowl, combine the cottage cheese, yogurt, chillies, coriander (if using), cumin and salt.

Spread 250 g (9 oz) of the salsa across the bottom of the baking dish. Arrange half of the tortillas evenly over the salsa. Spread half of the cheese mixture over the tortillas. Top with half of the beef or turkey mixture. Top with another 250 g (9 oz) of the salsa and 60 g (2 oz) of the grated cheese. Repeat the layering sequence with the remaining tortillas, cheese mixture and beef or turkey mixture. Sprinkle with the remaining salsa and cheese.

Bake for 30 minutes, or until heated through. Loosely cover with foil if the cheese browns too quickly.

Makes 8 servings

NUTRITION AT A GLANCE
Per serving: Energy 243 cals/1017 kJ; 10 g fat (of which 5 g saturates), 25 g protein, 15 g carbohydrate (of which 11 g sugars), 3 g fibre, 394 mg sodium

NORMAN'S

21 Almeria Avenue, Coral Gables, Florida

CHEF NORMAN VAN AKEN

THE MENU AT *NORMAN'S* FEATURES DISHES WITH AN INVENTIVE MIX OF FLAVOURS — A BLEND OF LATIN, NORTH AMERICAN, CARIBBEAN AND ASIAN — KNOWN AS NEW WORLD CUISINE. THESE TASTY PORK CHOPS ARE A PERFECT EXAMPLE.

Bolivian Spiced Pork Chops

PHASE 1

Split Peas

2½	tablespoons extra virgin olive oil
2	cloves garlic, finely chopped
½	onion, finely chopped
2	sticks of celery, finely chopped
1	carrot, finely chopped
1	teaspoon cayenne pepper
1	teaspoon ground cumin
1 L (1¾ pints)	chicken stock
1	smoked ham hock
1	bay leaf, broken in half
340 g (12 oz)	split peas

Pork Chops

1½	tablespoons ground cumin
3	teaspoons ground cardamom
3	teaspoons ground coriander
½	tablespoon cayenne pepper
3	tablespoons grated lemon zest
½	tablespoon sea salt
½	tablespoon ground black pepper
6	loin pork chops, each 4 cm (1½ in) thick, trimmed of all fat
3	tablespoons roasted garlic oil or extra virgin olive oil

To cook the peas: Heat the olive oil in a saucepan over medium–low heat. When hot, add the garlic and cook for 30 seconds. Turn up the heat to medium–high and add the onion, celery and carrot. When they start to turn golden, add the cayenne pepper and cumin. Stir and add the chicken stock, ham, bay leaf and split peas. Bring to a simmer, then turn down the heat and cook until the peas are tender, about 45 minutes. Remove and discard the bay leaf. Mash the split pea mixture. This will thicken as it cools.

To cook the pork: Preheat the oven to 180°C/350°F/gas 4.

In a small bowl, combine the cumin, cardamom, coriander, cayenne, lemon zest, salt and pepper. Put the pork chops in a sealable plastic bag. Sprinkle the spice mixture over the pork chops and rub it on both sides. Leave for 30 minutes

Heat a frying pan over medium–high heat. Add the oil and sear the chops on both sides. As they brown, put them on a baking sheet and finish them in the oven for 15 to 25 minutes, or until the juices run clear.

Note: I like to garnish this with sliced stuffed green olives and lemon wedges.

Makes 6 servings

NUTRITION AT A GLANCE
Per serving: Energy 508 cals/2126 kJ; 21 g fat (of which 5 g saturates), 45 g protein, 35 g carbohydrate (of which 3 g sugars), 3 g fibre, 579 mg sodium

Sage and Rosemary Pork

Ask your butcher to bone and butterfly the pork loin so it can be opened out, then rolled up evenly. The herb filling is a great way to infuse flavour into the meat, and this recipe is perfect when you're having guests for dinner.

Filling

- 2 tablespoons chopped fresh parsley
- 1½ tablespoons chopped fresh sage or thyme leaves
- 1 tablespoon chopped fresh rosemary
- 3 cloves garlic, finely chopped
- 3 tablespoons extra virgin olive oil
- 2 teaspoons Dijon mustard
- ¼ teaspoon salt
- ¼ teaspoon ground black pepper

Pork Loin

- 1 boneless pork loin joint (about 900 g/2 lb), butterflied
- ¾ teaspoon salt
- ½ teaspoon ground black pepper
- 1 tablespoon extra virgin olive oil
- sprigs of rosemary and sage, to garnish

To make the filling: In a small bowl, combine the parsley, sage or thyme, rosemary, garlic, oil, mustard, salt and pepper.

To cook the pork loin: Preheat the oven to 180°C/350°F/gas 4.

Sprinkle the inside of the pork loin with half of the salt and pepper. Spread the filling over the meat, leaving a 1 cm (½ in) border along one edge. Beginning at the opposite edge, roll the loin up to wrap the filling. Using kitchen string, tie the loin every 4 cm (1½ in) to hold its shape.

Rub the loin with the oil and sprinkle with the remaining salt and pepper. Place the meat in a roasting tin and roast in the centre of the oven for 1 hour, or until a thermometer inserted in the centre registers 70C°/155°F and the juices run clear. Leave to stand for 10 minutes before carving.

To prevent slices from unrolling, skewer the roast every 5 mm (¼ in) with wooden cocktail sticks along the edge where the roll ends. Slice crosswise between the cocktail sticks and ties. Remove the string before serving. Garnish with the sage and rosemary sprigs.

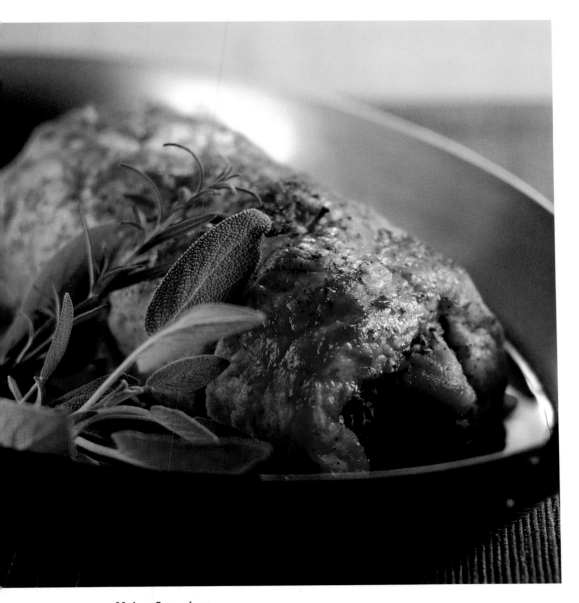

Makes 6 servings

Timo (Italian for thyme) is a handsome bistro co-owned by acclaimed chef Tim Andriola. *Timo's* menu spotlights Andriola's flair and appreciation for the flavours of Italy and the Mediterranean.

Roasted Pork Tenderloin with Chickpeas, Roasted Peppers and Clams

PHASE 2

120 ml (4 fl oz) orange juice

1 tablespoon lime juice

6 tablespoons rapeseed (canola) oil

2 tablespoons wholegrain mustard

1 tablespoon chopped garlic

½ tablespoon paprika

1 tablespoon chopped fresh thyme leaves

½ tablespoon black peppercorns

1 whole pork tenderloin (about 400–455 g/ 14 oz–1 lb), trimmed of all visible fat

salt and pepper

1 tablespoon finely chopped shallot

1 head garlic

1 small red + 1 small yellow pepper (capsicum), roasted, skin and seeds removed, chopped

2 tomatoes, skinned, seeded and chopped

200 g (7 oz) cooked chickpeas

180 ml (6 fl oz) chicken stock

12 fresh clams

1 tablespoon chopped fresh parsley

In a large bowl, combine the orange juice, lime juice, 4 tablespoons of the oil, the mustard, chopped garlic, paprika, thyme and peppercorns. Submerge the pork in this marinade for at least 6 to 8 hours, preferably overnight.

Remove the pork from the marinade and pat dry with paper towels. Season with the salt and pepper.

Preheat the oven to 180°C/350°F/gas 4.

Heat the remaining 2 tablespoons oil in an ovenproof heavy sauté pan over medium-high heat. Sauté the shallot and garlic for 3 to 5 minutes, until lightly browned. Add the pork, brown evenly and then place in the oven for 10 to 15 minutes.

Remove the pan from the oven. Remove the pork from the pan and leave in a warm place to rest for a few minutes.

In the same sauté pan over medium heat, add the peppers, tomatoes, chickpeas and stock and bring to a simmer. Add the clams and cover the pan tightly. When the clams open, transfer them to 4 serving plates. Add the parsley to the pan and adjust the seasoning with salt and pepper. Spoon the chickpea mixture into the centre of the plates. Slice the pork into thin slices and arrange on top of the chickpeas.

Makes 4 servings

NUTRITION AT A GLANCE
Per serving: Energy 454 cals/1900 kJ; 27 g fat (of which 5 g saturates), 34 g protein, 20 g carbohydrate (of which 10 g sugars), 4 g fibre, 749 mg sodium

Garlic and Soy Grilled Pork

Grill or barbecue chunks of vegetables alongside this lip-smacking pork for an irresistible feast. Red and yellow peppers (capsicums), onion and courgette (zucchini) would work well.

4 boneless pork loin chops, trimmed of all visible fat

1 tablespoon light soy sauce

2 teaspoons finely chopped garlic

½ teaspoon paprika

½ teaspoon salt

¼ teaspoon ground black pepper

 fresh herbs, to garnish

Sprinkle the pork all over with soy sauce, garlic, paprika, salt and pepper. Cover and refrigerate at least 20 minutes, or up to 2 hours.

Coat a grill rack or ridged grilling pan with cooking spray. Preheat the grill or pan.

Cook the pork for 10 to 12 minutes, turning halfway through cooking time, or until a thermometer inserted in the centre of the meat registers 70C°/155°F and the juices run clear. Garnish with the herbs.

Makes 4 servings

NUTRITION AT A GLANCE

Per serving: Energy 226 cals/946 kJ; 10 g fat (of which 3 g saturates), 32 g protein, 1 g carbohydrate (of which 0 g sugars), 0 g fibre, 620 mg sodium

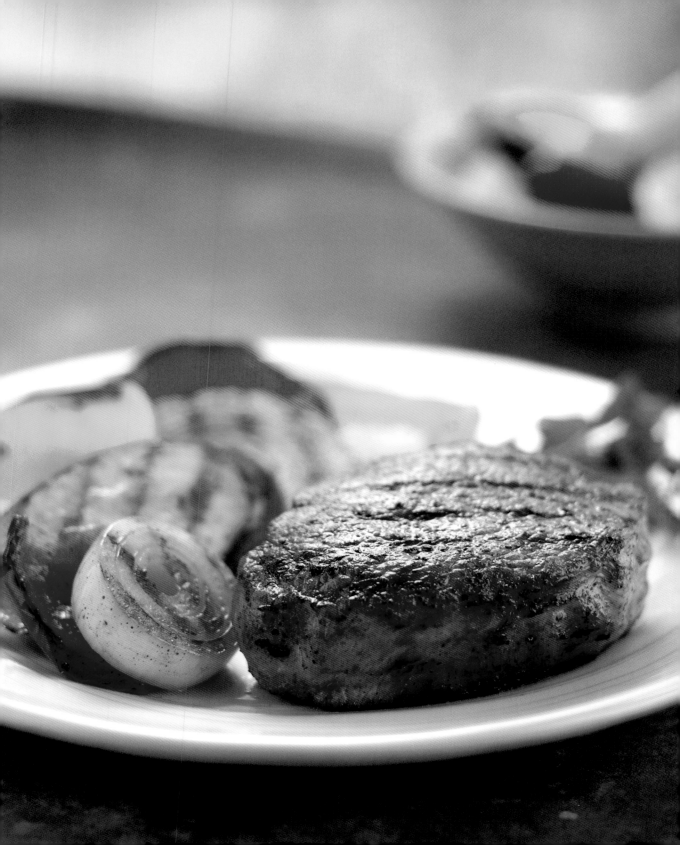

From the Menu of . . .

BLUE DOOR AT DELANO

1685 Collins Avenue, Miami Beach, Florida

CHEF CLAUDE TROISGROS

LOCATED IN THE DELANO HOTEL, ONE OF MIAMI BEACH'S
HIP HOTELS, *BLUE DOOR AT DELANO* WAS NAMED ONE OF AMERICA'S
BEST NEW RESTAURANTS OF 1998 BY *ESQUIRE* MAGAZINE.
IN A CHIC, ART DECO SETTING, CONSULTING CHEF CLAUDE TROISGROS
HAS TEAMED WITH CHEF DAMON GORDON TO PRODUCE MODERN,
FRENCH–BASED CUISINE WITH A TROPICAL INFLUENCE.

Veal Mignon

PHASE 3

8	baby artichokes	
60 g (2 oz)	shallots, chopped	
5	cloves chopped garlic	
5	tablespoons extra virgin olive oil	
4	tablespoons soy sauce	
12	medallions of veal (about 75 g/2½ oz each)	

30 g (1 oz)	sun-dried tomatoes, cut into thin strips
5	tablespoons capers
5	tablespoons raisins
	chopped parsley
	salt
	pepper
	fresh thyme (optional)

In a saucepan, cook the artichokes in boiling water until tender, about 20 minutes. Leave to cool. Remove the top and outer leaves; cut the artichokes into quarters.

In a sauté pan, lightly sauté the shallots and garlic in 3 tablespoons of the olive oil until tender. Add the soy sauce and simmer until slightly reduced. Remove the sauce from the pan and set aside.

Add the remaining 2 tablespoons of olive oil to the sauté pan and sauté the veal until medium-rare. Transfer the veal to a warm platter. In the same pan, sauté the artichokes, sun-dried tomatoes, capers and raisins. Sprinkle with chopped parsley and season with salt and pepper to taste.

Place 3 pieces of veal on each plate, add the artichoke mixture and spoon the sauce over the top. Garnish with the thyme, if using.

Makes 4 servings

NUTRITION AT A GLANCE
Per serving: Energy 504 cals/2110 kJ; 19 g fat (of which 4.5 g saturates), 52 g protein, 32 g carbohydrate (of which 29 g sugars), 3 g fibre, 1412 mg sodium

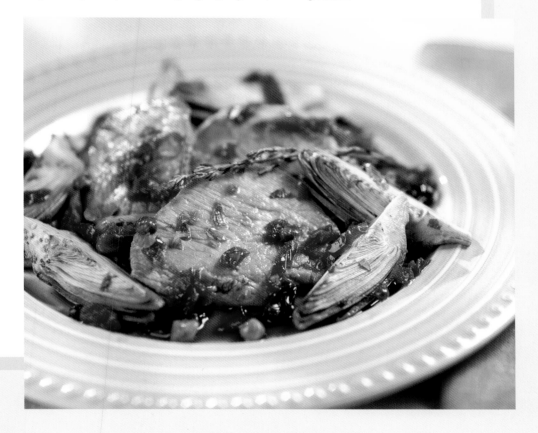

Sesame Pork Tenderloin

The sesame seeds give the pork a mild, nutty flavour.

2	lean pork tenderloins (about 340–455 g/12 oz–1 lb each)
4	tablespoons extra virgin olive oil
4	tablespoons sesame seeds
1	stick of celery, chopped
2	tablespoons chopped onion
45 g (1½ oz)	fresh wholemeal breadcrumbs
1	teaspoon lemon juice
1	teaspoon Worcestershire sauce
½	teaspoon salt
½	teaspoon dried thyme
⅛	teaspoon ground black pepper

Preheat the oven to 160°C/325°F/gas 3.

Cut each tenderloin almost through lengthwise, then place between two sheets of greaseproof paper and beat with a meat mallet to flatten.

Heat the oil in a large frying pan over medium-high heat. Add the sesame seeds, celery and onion and cook, stirring frequently, for 3 minutes, or until lightly browned. Add the breadcrumbs, lemon juice, Worcestershire sauce, salt, thyme and pepper. Toss lightly to mix. Spread the stuffing on the cut surface of one tenderloin. Place the second tenderloin cut side down on top of the stuffing. Fasten the tenderloins together with kitchen string or skewers. Coat a roasting tin with cooking spray and place the pork in the tin.

Roast for 1 hour and 20 minutes, or until a thermometer inserted in the centre registers 70°C/155°F and the juices run clear. Leave to stand for 10 minutes before slicing.

Makes 6 servings

NUTRITION AT A GLANCE
Per serving: Energy 330 cals/1381 kJ; 21 g fat (of which 5 g saturates), 30 g protein, 4 g carbohydrate (of which 1 g sugars), 1 g fibre, 389 mg sodium

MY SOUTH BEACH DIET

FOR THE FIRST TIME, I TRULY UNDERSTAND 'EAT TO LIVE, NOT LIVE TO EAT'.

I reached my highest weight ever last year at 112 kg (17½ st). On top of that, I was taking medication for high blood pressure, arthritis and anxiety, as well as a painkiller for PMS symptoms. I felt horrible, frequently called in sick to work and looked awful, wearing anything that would cover the fat. I was moody, irritable and depressed, which took a toll on my husband and three children.

I started to walk around the shopping centre and in five months I lost 4.5 kg (10 lb). It was a good start, and I began to feel better. But I hadn't changed my eating habits. Everything I read seemed too hard, too time-consuming, or too expensive. I'd tried many weight loss plans and numerous fad diets. I never stuck with anything. They just didn't work for me with full-time work and mothering.

When a magazine featuring the South Beach Diet arrived, it literally started a new life for me. After Phase 1, when you 'detox' your body, I noticed a huge change in my taste buds. I crave salads now and find them very satisfying. Yogurt tastes extremely sweet and satisfies my sweet tooth. For the first time, I'm really tasting my food and feeling satisfied with a different palate of foods. My cravings for pasta, pastries and bread have completely disappeared.

So far I'm down to 92 kg (14½ st), well on my way to my goal of under 64 kg (10 st). My clothing size has dropped from a size 24 to a size 18. My blood pressure and arthritis medication has been adjusted to almost half of what I was taking. Another positive side effect has been a reduction of the severe PMS symptoms I had been experiencing – surely a combination of the soy I have added to my diet and my new South Beach way of life.

Throughout my weight loss, my family has been so supportive. My 14-year-old is amazed to be able to feel my ribs. My 7-year-old asks, 'Can you eat this?' and I respond, 'Yes, I could have that, but I'd really rather have this, because it's healthier.' She's getting the message early about making better choices. My husband has been wonderful, too, cooking meals when I say I need to go for a walk, which I now do three times a week, for 3 to 5 miles.

For the first time, I truly understand the expression 'Eat to live, not live to eat'. Understanding this is what really changed my mind-set, not to mention my appearance. *–TERRI L.*

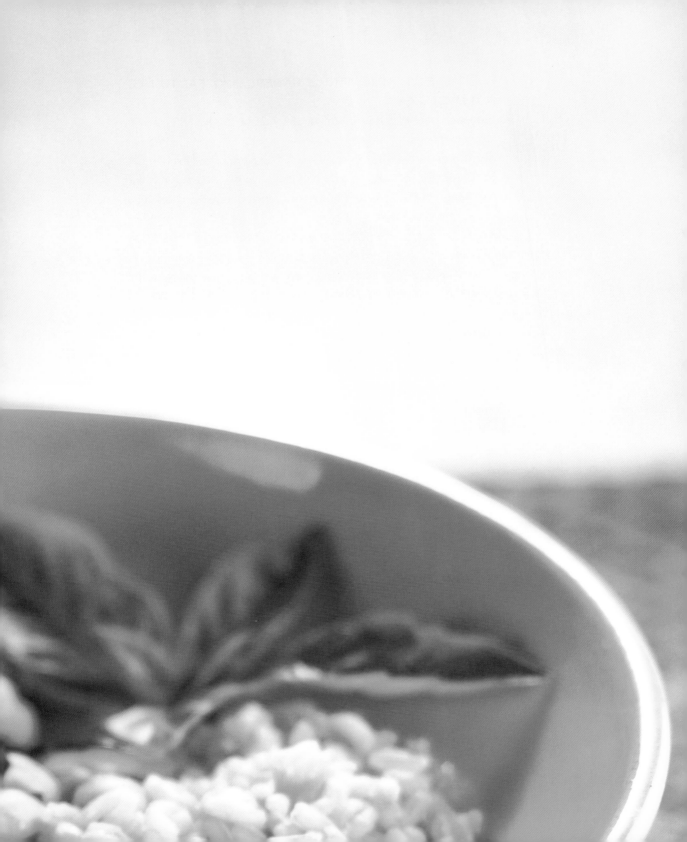

VEGETARIAN DISHES

EVEN VEGETARIANS SOMETIMES NEED HELP WITH WEIGHT CONTROL. WHEN YOU'RE NOT GETTING PROTEIN FROM MEAT, YOU TEND TO RELY MORE HEAVILY ON CARBOHYDRATES, WHICH CAN LEAD TO OVER-INDULGING IN SOME OF THE WRONG KINDS. BUT YOU CAN EAT WELL ON THE SOUTH BEACH DIET EVEN IF YOU DON'T INCLUDE FISH OR MEAT IN THE PLAN.

TOFU, MADE FROM SOYA BEANS, IS A TERRIFIC STAPLE OF THE VEGETARIAN DIET. IT'S A GREAT SOURCE OF PROTEIN AND CAN BE THE FOCUS OF EXTREMELY TASTY DISHES. THE BEAUTY OF TOFU IS HOW IT TAKES ON THE FLAVOUR OF WHATEVER SEASONINGS YOU USE, AS IN OUR RECIPE FOR STIR-FRY OF BROCCOLI WITH TOFU AND CHERRY TOMATOES.

BEANS, CHICKPEAS AND LENTILS ARE ALL ALLOWED IN PHASE 1. IN PHASE 2 YOU CAN REINTRODUCE WHOLE GRAINS, SUCH AS BARLEY AND BROWN RICE, AS WELL AS PASTA MADE FROM WHOLE WHEAT OR SPELT, AN ANCIENT CEREAL GRAIN THAT'S RICH IN PROTEIN.

Thai Vegetables in Coconut Milk

An authentic Thai dish has five flavour elements: hot/spicy, salty, sweet, bitter/aromatic and sour.

400 ml (14 fl oz)	reduced-fat (no sugar added) coconut milk
2	cloves garlic, chopped
½	teaspoon grated lemon zest
½	teaspoon grated lime zest
250 g (9 oz)	asparagus tips, sliced
90 g (3 oz)	mushrooms, halved
1	small red pepper (capsicum), sliced
1	small head pak choi (bok choy), stems sliced and leaves left whole
40 g (1¼ oz)	unsalted peanuts
½	teaspoon dried chilli flakes
1	tablespoon light soy sauce
1	tablespoon fresh lime juice
1	tablespoon fresh lemon juice
1	small bunch fresh basil, shredded

In a food processor, combine the coconut milk, garlic, lemon zest and lime zest. Pulse to process into a paste. Transfer to a large frying pan, place over medium–high heat and cook, stirring, for 1 minute. Add the asparagus, mushrooms, red pepper, pak choi, peanuts and chilli flakes and simmer for 10 minutes.

Stir in the soy sauce, lime juice, lemon juice and basil and simmer, stirring constantly, for 5 minutes. Serve hot.

Makes 4 servings

NUTRITION AT A GLANCE
Per serving: Energy 173 cals/724 kJ; 7 g fat (of which 2 g saturates), 11 g protein, 16 g carbohydrate (of which 14 g sugars), 5 g fibre, 280 mg sodium

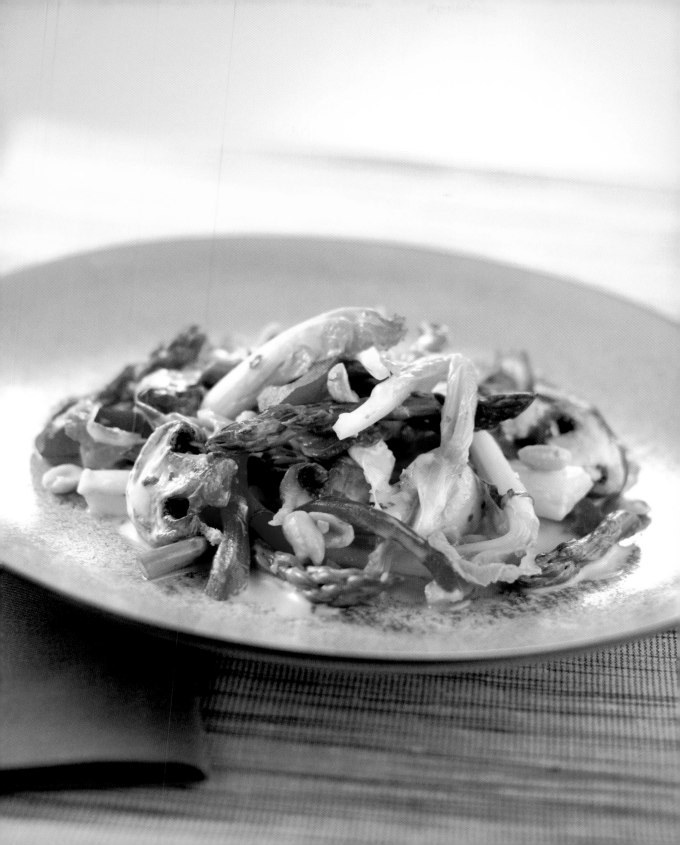

Chickpea Basil Sauté

Chickpeas have been a staple of the Orient and Mediterranean for centuries. They are an excellent source of protein and fibre. This makes a great vegetarian main course — or serve as an accompaniment to one of the chicken recipes. Without the brown rice, this is a Phase 1 recipe.

1	tablespoon extra virgin olive oil
2	onions, sliced
½	teaspoon cumin seeds
1	small red pepper (capsicum), cut into strips
1	tablespoon water
3	spring onions, chopped
2 × 400 g (14 oz)	tins chickpeas, rinsed and drained
2	bunches fresh basil, chopped
170 g (6 oz)	brown rice, cooked and kept hot
	sprigs of basil, to garnish

Heat the oil in a large non-stick frying pan over medium-high heat. Add the onions and cumin seeds and cook, stirring frequently, for 7 minutes. Add the red pepper and water. Cover, reduce the heat to low and cook for 2 minutes. Add the spring onions and chickpeas and cook for 2 minutes. Remove from the heat and add the basil. Serve with the rice and garnish with sprigs of basil.

Makes 4 servings

NUTRITION AT A GLANCE

Per serving: Energy 330 cals/1380 kJ; 8 g fat (of which 1 g saturates), 14 g protein, 52 g carbohydrate (of which 8 g sugars), 6 g fibre, 320 mg sodium

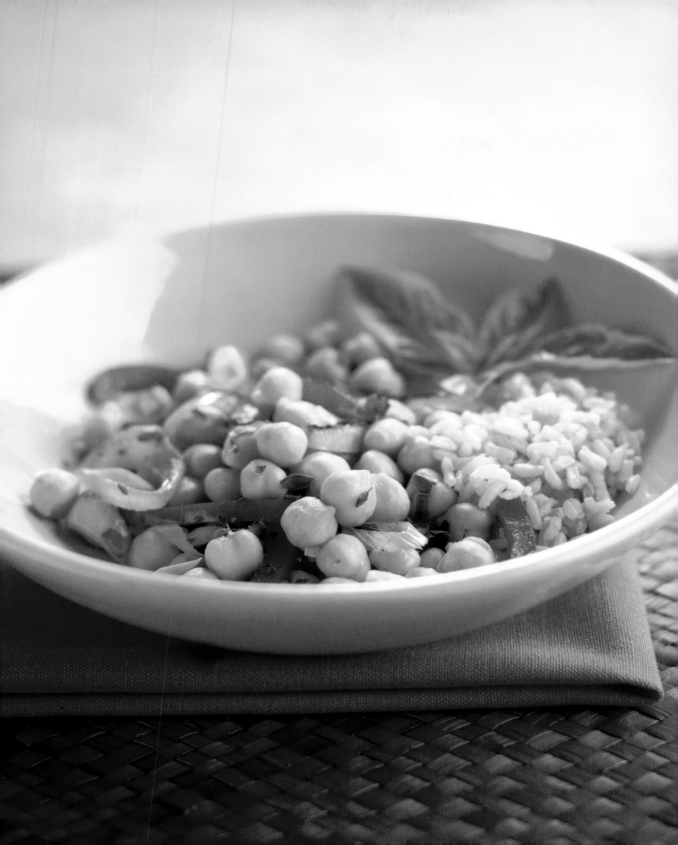

BLEAU VIEW, FONTAINEBLEAU HILTON RESORT

4441 Collins Avenue, Miami Beach, Florida

CHEF BILL ZUPPAS

LOCATED AT ONE OF MIAMI'S BEST-LOVED RESORTS, THE *BLEAU VIEW* COMBINES EUROPEAN AMBIANCE WITH SOUTH BEACH STYLE. THE UPDATED CONTINENTAL FARE, LIKE THIS RISOTTO, RELIES HEAVILY ON MEDITERRANEAN FLAVOURS AND SPICES.

Mediterranean Vegetable Risotto

PHASE 2

375 g (13 oz) organic short-grain brown rice	2 carrots, chopped
1 L (1¾ pints) water	2 sticks of celery, trimmed and chopped
3 tablespoons extra virgin olive oil	1 large tomato, seeded and chopped
230 g (8 oz) green beans, cut into 1 cm (½ in) pieces	2 tablespoons chopped fresh parsley
200 g (7 oz) green cabbage, shredded	sea salt
1 onion, finely chopped	freshly ground black pepper
1 clove garlic, finely chopped	

Put the rice, water and 1 tablespoon of the oil in a saucepan with a tightly fitting lid. Bring to the boil, reduce the heat, cover and simmer for 50 minutes. Remove from the heat and leave to stand, covered, for 10 minutes.

Meanwhile, bring a saucepan of water to the boil and cook the beans for 3 to 4 minutes, or until tender. Add the cabbage and cook for 2 to 3 minutes, or until tender. Drain the vegetables and set aside.

Heat the remaining 2 tablespoons of oil in a large frying pan. Sauté the onion, garlic, carrots and celery until crisp-tender.

Add the tomato, green beans and cabbage and heat through.

Add the rice and heat through. Remove from the heat and stir in the parsley. Season with salt and pepper to taste.

Makes 8 (side dish) servings

NUTRITION AT A GLANCE
Per serving: Energy 235 cals/984 kJ; 6 g fat (of which 1 g saturates), 5 g protein, 44 g carbohydrate (of which 5 g sugars), 3 g fibre, 160 mg sodium

Tofu alla Cacciatora

Alla cacciatora means 'hunter-style'. Because I'm not a hunter, I decided to take solace after a hard day's hunt (work) with tofu instead of pheasant or hare.

455 g (1 lb) firm tofu, cut into 1 cm (½ in) slices

½ onion, sliced

½ red pepper (capsicum), sliced

½ green pepper (capsicum), sliced

2 tablespoons white wine

1 large clove garlic, finely chopped

1 teaspoon dried basil

1 teaspoon dried oregano

pinch of allspice

2 × 400 g (14 oz) tins tomatoes (400 g/14 oz), drained

2 teaspoons tomato purée (concentrate

sprigs of rosemary, to garnish

Cover a 43 × 28 cm (17 in × 11 in) baking sheet with paper towels. Place the tofu in a single layer on the towels. Cover the tofu with paper towels and pat down on the tofu until dry. Discard all the paper towels and rearrange the tofu in a single layer on the baking sheet.

Preheat the oven to 180°C/350°F/gas 4.

Coat a large frying pan with olive oil cooking spray and place over medium heat. Add the onion and peppers and cook, stirring frequently, for 5 minutes. Add the wine, garlic, basil, oregano and allspice and cook, stirring, for 1 minute. Add the tomatoes and tomato purée. Bring to the boil and simmer for 15 minutes.

Coat another large frying pan with olive oil cooking spray and place over medium heat. Add the tofu and sauté for 3 minutes, or until lightly browned on both sides. Place the browned tofu slices in a baking dish and cover with the tomato sauce.

Bake for 1 hour, or until cooked through. Garnish with the rosemary.

Makes 4 servings

NUTRITION AT A GLANCE

Per serving: Energy 133 cals/556 kJ; 5 g fat (of which 0.5 g saturates), 11 g protein, 10 g carbohydrate (of which 8 g sugars), 2 g fibre, 500 mg sodium

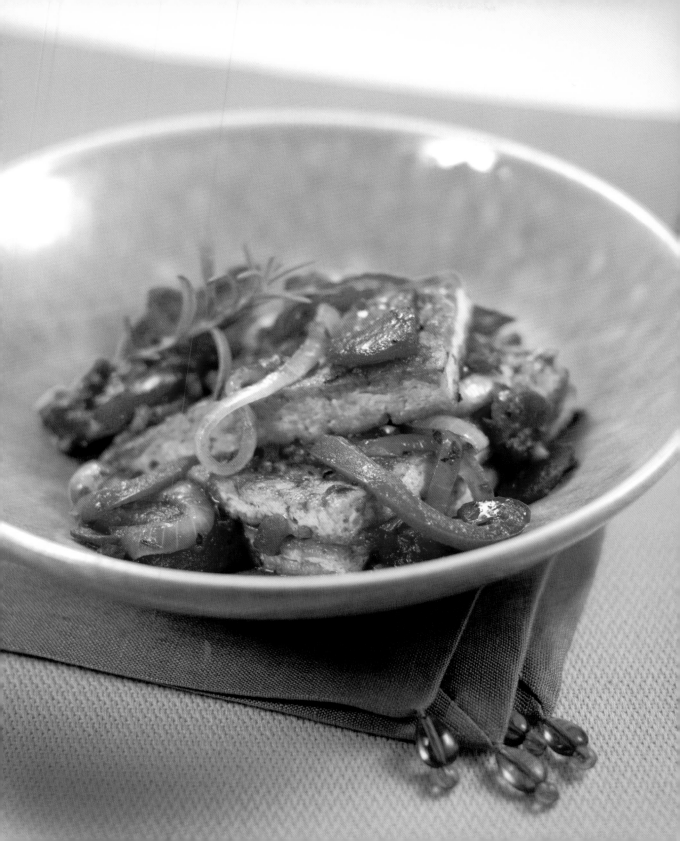

Stir-Fry of Broccoli with Tofu and Cherry Tomatoes

Tofu is a chameleon ingredient that takes on the flavours of the foods that it cooks with. Here, it adopts a sweet-and-sour flavour from garlic, sherry and soy sauce. Stir-fries cook very quickly, so be sure to have all your ingredients chopped and ready to add to the pan before you begin cooking.

80 ml (3 fl oz)	vegetable stock
1	tablespoon light soy sauce
1	tablespoon dry sherry
2	tablespoons cornflour
1	tablespoon rapeseed (canola) oil
1	large bunch broccoli, cut into small florets
4	cloves garlic, finely chopped
1	tablespoon finely chopped fresh ginger
115 g (4 oz)	mushrooms, sliced
145 g (5 oz)	red or yellow cherry tomatoes, halved
230 g (8 oz)	firm tofu, drained and cut into 5 mm (¼ in) cubes

In a cup, whisk together the stock, soy sauce, sherry and cornflour. Set aside.

Heat the oil in a large non-stick frying pan over medium–high heat. Add the broccoli, garlic and ginger and cook, stirring constantly, for 1 minute. Add the mushrooms and cook, stirring frequently, for 3 minutes, or until tender and lightly browned.

Add the tomatoes and tofu and cook, stirring frequently, for 2 minutes, or until the tomatoes begin to collapse.

Stir the cornflour mixture and add to the pan. Cook, stirring, for 2 minutes, or until the mixture boils and thickens. Serve immediately.

Makes 4 servings

NUTRITION AT A GLANCE
Per serving: Energy 164 cals/686 kJ; 6 g fat (of which 1 g saturates), 10 g protein, 16 g carbohydrate (of which 3 g sugars), 3 g fibre, 235 mg sodium

Tofu with Salsa

The habañero chilli gives you lots of flavour — and quite a bit of heat. Smoked tofu is one of the tastiest of tofu products, but each brand tastes different, so experiment to see which one you like the best.

230 g (8 oz) smoked tofu, cut into 8 thin slices

1 large beefsteak tomato, skinned, seeded and finely chopped

4 tablespoons extra virgin olive oil

1 clove garlic, finely chopped

2 tablespoons chopped fresh parsley

1 small habañero (very hot red) chilli, seeded and finely chopped (wear rubber gloves when handling)

1 teaspoon red wine vinegar

¼ teaspoon sugar substitute

Place the tofu in a single layer in a shallow dish.

In a small bowl combine the tomato, oil, garlic, parsley, chilli, vinegar and sugar substitute and mix well.

Spoon the salsa mixture over the tofu and leave to marinate for 30 minutes.

Serve 2 slices of tofu on each plate, topped with the salsa.

Makes 4 servings

NUTRITION AT A GLANCE
Per serving: Energy 175 cals/732 kJ; 15 g fat (of which 3 g saturates), 8 g protein, 3 g carbohydrate (of which 1 g sugars), 0.5 g fibre, 250 mg sodium

From the Menu of . . .

CHEF ALLEN'S

19088 NE 29th Avenue, Aventura, Florida

CHEF-PROPRIETOR ALLEN SUSSER

BEFITTING ITS SUNNY SOUTH FLORIDA LOCATION, *CHEF ALLEN'S* SERVES WHAT
CHEF-PROPRIETOR ALLEN SUSSER CALLS 'PALM TREE CUISINE'. IT'S A
KIND OF GLOBAL THINKING ABOUT FOOD AND RECIPES THAT, AS HE PUTS IT,
'ENCOURAGES THE FUSING OF INGREDIENTS OF MANY CUISINES AND CULTURES.'

Caribbean Ratatouille

PHASE 3

2	tablespoons extra virgin olive oil
1	large onion, chopped
1	small green plantain, chopped
145 g (5 oz)	calabaza, acorn squash or butternut squash, chopped
2	medium chayote (see p.137) or courgettes (zucchini), chopped
2	medium Anaheim (mild green) chillies, seeded and chopped
1	medium red pepper (capsicum), seeded and chopped
½	tablespoon chopped garlic
1	teaspoon dried oregano
1	teaspoon ground cumin
1	teaspoon ground black peppercorns
1	tablespoon sea salt
240 ml (8 fl oz)	freshly squeezed orange juice

In a large casserole dish, warm the olive oil. Add the onion and cook until translucent. Then add each of the vegetables at 2-minute intervals, starting with the plantain, then the squash, chayote, chilli and red pepper. Stir well but try not to crush any of the vegetables.

Season with the garlic, oregano, cumin, peppercorns and salt. Moisten the mixture with orange juice. Simmer for 5 minutes, or until tender, allowing all the flavours to unite yet not losing the integrity of each vegetable.

Note: calabaza is a green pumpkin, sometimes available from West Indian shops.

Makes 4 servings

NUTRITION AT A GLANCE
Per serving: Energy 150 cals/628 kJ; 6 g fat (of which 1 g saturates), 2 g protein, 14 g carbohydrate (of which 11 g sugars), 2 g fibre, 1461 mg sodium

Spinach Dumplings

These light dumplings are a South Beach version of the Italian gnocchi verdi.

455 g (1 lb)	frozen chopped spinach
2	teaspoons salt
2	eggs
75 g (2½ oz)	fresh wholemeal breadcrumbs
1	teaspoon Italian herb seasoning
300 g (10½ oz)	ricotta cheese (reduced-fat if available)
30 g (1 oz)	Parmesan cheese, grated
3	spring onions, finely chopped
5	tablespoons chopped fresh parsley
2	teaspoons finely chopped fresh basil
1	clove garlic, finely chopped
	pinch of ground nutmeg
	pinch of ground black pepper
	wholemeal flour
	South Beach Tomato Sauce (see page 156)

Put the spinach and 1½ teaspoons of the salt in a saucepan over low heat, cover and cook for 15 minutes, or until the spinach is completely thawed. Drain. Use your hands to squeeze out as much water as possible.

Beat the eggs in a large bowl. Add the spinach, breadcrumbs, Italian seasoning, ricotta, Parmesan, spring onions, parsley, basil, garlic, nutmeg and pepper. Mix well, then cover and refrigerate for 24 hours.

Preheat the oven to 120°C/250°F/gas ½. Coat an ovenproof dish with olive oil cooking spray.

Form the spinach mixture into oval dumplings, about 8 cm (3 in) long and 4 cm (1½ in) wide. Roll each dumpling in flour. Do not allow the dumplings to touch each other as you finish them.

Bring 4–6 litres (7–10 pints) water and the remaining ½ teaspoon salt to the boil in a large saucepan over medium-high heat. Drop enough dumplings into the water to make one layer. When the dumplings float to the surface, cook for an additional 4 minutes. Remove the dumplings with a slotted spoon, draining well.

Place the dumplings in the prepared dish and place in the oven to keep warm. Cook the remaining dumplings in the same manner. When all the dumplings are in the oven, warm the tomato sauce in a saucepan over medium-low heat.

Divide the dumplings among 4 serving dishes and top with a little of the tomato sauce. Serve additional sauce on the side.

Makes 4 servings

NUTRITION AT A GLANCE
Per serving: Energy 330 cals/1380 kJ; 20 g fat (of which 10 g saturates), 20 g protein, 18 g carbohydrate (of which 6 g sugars), 5 g fibre, 1659 mg sodium

Rocket and Basil Pesto Linguine

Spelt is a high-protein ancient grain that's enjoying a resurgence. If you can't find spelt pasta in the supermarket or health food shop, use wholewheat linguine or spaghetti. This tasty dish is perfect for supper on a cold night.

340 g (12 oz)	spelt linguine
75 g (2½ oz)	rocket
45 g (1½ oz)	basil leaves
3–4	cloves garlic, finely chopped
2	tablespoons pine nuts
	salt
	freshly ground black pepper
5	tablespoons extra virgin olive oil
30 g (1 oz)	Parmesan cheese, grated

Cook the pasta according to package directions. Drain and place in a large serving bowl.

Meanwhile, in a food processor, combine the rocket, basil, garlic, pine nuts and salt and pepper to taste. Process to chop coarsely.

With the food processor running, slowly add the oil in a steady stream until the mixture is smooth.

Toss the pasta with the pesto, sprinkle with the cheese and serve hot.

Makes 4 servings

NUTRITION AT A GLANCE
Per serving: Energy 511 cals/2139 kJ; 25 g fat (of which 4 g saturates), 17 g protein, 58 g carbohydrate (of which 4 g sugars), 8 g fibre, 396 mg sodium

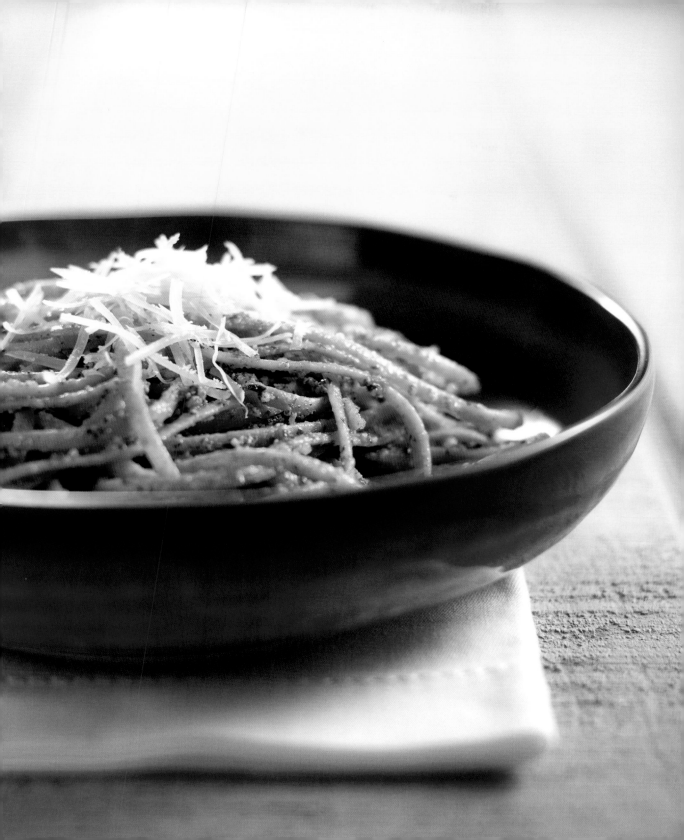

Vegetable Lasagne

This dish can be enjoyed right away, but it tastes even better the next day.

1	teaspoon extra virgin olive oil
1	courgette (zucchini), sliced
455 g (1 lb)	ricotta cheese (reduced-fat if available)
1	egg
2	tablespoons chopped fresh basil
¼	teaspoon salt
⅛	teaspoon ground black pepper
450 ml (15 fl oz)	South Beach Tomato Sauce (see page 156) or low-sugar pasta sauce
9	wholewheat lasagne sheets, cooked
285 g (10 oz)	frozen chopped spinach, thawed and squeezed dry
30 g (1 oz)	Parmesan cheese, grated
30 g (1 oz)	reduced-fat mozzarella cheese, grated

Preheat the oven to 180°C/350°F/gas 4. Coat a 32 × 23 cm (13 × 9 in) baking dish with cooking spray.

Heat the oil in a frying pan over medium heat. Add the courgette and cook for 5 minutes, or until just tender. Remove from the heat and set aside.

In a bowl, combine the ricotta, egg, basil, salt and pepper. Set aside a quarter of the tomato sauce.

Place 3 sheets of lasagne in the prepared baking dish. Spoon half of the remaining tomato sauce over the lasagne. Top with half of the ricotta mixture, half of the spinach, half of the courgette and half of the Parmesan. Repeat layering with 3 more sheets of lasagne and the remaining ingredients. Cover with the remaining 3 sheets of lasagne. Spoon the reserved sauce over the top and sprinkle with the mozzarella.

Cover with foil and bake for 25 minutes. Remove the foil and bake for a further 20 minutes, or until hot and bubbling. Leave to stand for 10 minutes before serving.

Makes 8 servings

NUTRITION AT A GLANCE

Per serving: Energy 281 cals/1176 kJ; 15 g fat (of which 7 g saturates), 14 g protein, 24 g carbohydrate (of which 5 g sugars), 4 g fibre, 401 mg sodium

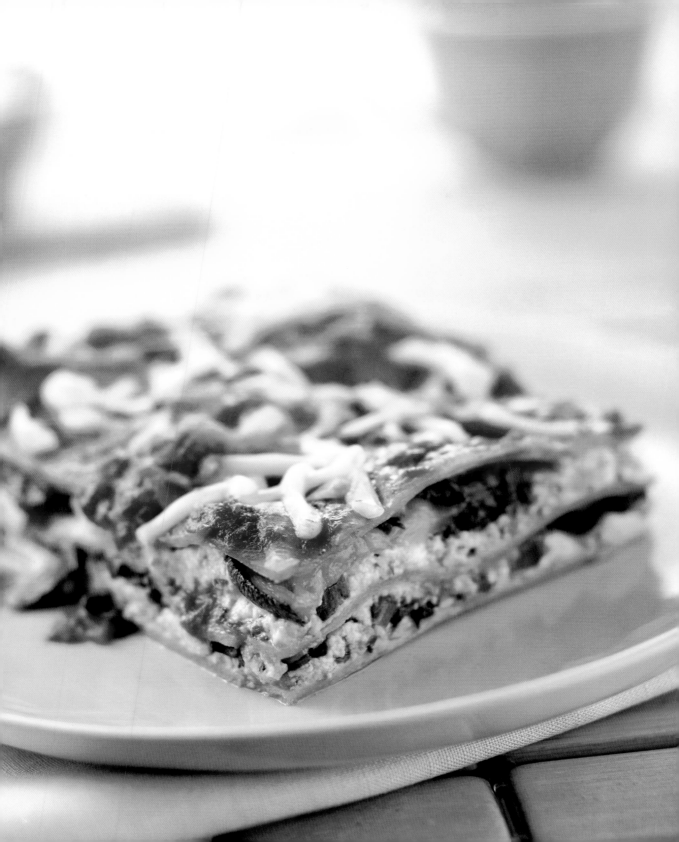

Vegetarian Chilli with Avocado Salsa

This flavour-packed chilli will leave you wondering where you could put any meat, even if you wanted it.

Avocado Salsa

1 ripe avocado, peeled, pitted and finely chopped

1 small tomato, finely chopped

¼ red onion, finely chopped

1 clove garlic, finely chopped

1 tablespoon chopped fresh coriander

juice of 1 large lime

¼ teaspoon ground cumin

¼ teaspoon ground black pepper

Vegetarian Chilli

2 teaspoons extra virgin olive oil

1 onion, chopped

1 red pepper (capsicum), chopped

400 g (14 oz) tinned black beans or red kidney beans, drained and rinsed

400 g (14 oz) tinned chopped tomatoes

300 ml (10 fl oz) vegetable stock

1–2 green chillies, chopped

2 teaspoons chilli powder

2 cloves garlic, finely chopped

1 teaspoon ground cumin

1 teaspoon dried oregano

4 tablespoons fat-free natural yogurt

1 lime, cut into 6 wedges

2 tablespoons chopped fresh coriander

To make the avocado salsa: In a large bowl, combine the avocado, tomato, onion, garlic, coriander, lime juice, cumin and pepper. Mix gently. Leave to stand for 30 minutes.

To make the chilli: Heat the oil in a large casserole over medium–high heat. Add the onion and pepper and cook, stirring frequently, for 3 minutes. Add the beans, tomatoes (with juice), stock, chillies, chilli powder, garlic, cumin and oregano and simmer for 20 minutes.

Serve the chilli with the avocado salsa, yogurt and lime wedges. Sprinkle with the coriander.

Makes 6 servings

NUTRITION AT A GLANCE
Per serving: Energy 180 cals/753 kJ; 8 g fat (of which 2 g saturates), 8 g protein, 20 g carbohydrate (of which 10 g sugars), 6 g fibre, 397 mg sodium

MY SOUTH BEACH DIET

I'M FOCUSING ON MAKING MEALS THAT ARE AESTHETICALLY PLEASING AND BEAUTIFUL TO LOOK AT.

I'm 47 years old and single. I'd always enjoyed a healthy, active lifestyle and felt great until last year, when an unexpected hysterectomy got me off track emotionally and physically. I stopped exercising, ate the wrong things, and gained about 22 kg (3½ st) while recovering from surgery. My doctor made it clear that if I didn't start making changes, I was headed towards diabetes.

I started with a weight-loss support group. It was convenient because we had weekly meetings at work. Then I heard about South Beach, and now I am doing a kind of hybrid approach: eating the South Beach way, and receiving emotional support through the group.

I've lost 27 kg (more than 4 st) so far, but have not yet reached my goal of wearing clothes smaller than a size 14. For me, slow and steady has been key. I like the structure of the SB plan. Deprivation leads to bingeing, in my experience, and this diet allows you the things you want. Before South Beach, I was the kind of person who could eat a whole loaf of French bread. Now I can have a piece of French bread if I want to, but my meals are more balanced.

Another thing that has helped is focusing on making meals that are aesthetically pleasing and beautiful to look at. I've become very fond of vegetables – their colours and textures are amazing! I'm more visually aware of food. When I've created something beautiful to look at, I savour it – no more cramming!

Eating out is often a challenge, but I have found that telling people I have dietary restrictions garners more respect than saying I am on a diet. I am not shy about asking for substitutions, and I ask that waiting staff bring a takeaway container to the table when they bring the meal, so that I can save half for later.

For me, weight control has shifted from wanting to be model-thin or attract a certain type of man, to wanting to maintain a healthy BMI (body mass index), to avoid obesity-related conditions such as diabetes, and to live a long life. Life is a gift, and keeping myself in shape is the best gift that I can give to myself.

– SUSAN W.

From the Menu of . . .

MACALUSO'S

1747 Alton Road, Miami Beach, Florida

CHEF MICHAEL D'ANDREA

ESCAROLE AND BEANS IS A CLASSIC ITALIAN DISH THAT'S RIGHT AT HOME AT THIS FRIENDLY TRATTORIA, A FAVOURITE OF MIAMI BEACH LOCALS.

Macaluso's Escarole and Beans

PHASE 1

4 tablespoons extra virgin olive oil	3 heads escarole (Batavian endive), cut into 5–8 cm (2–3 in) pieces
5 cloves garlic, finely chopped	
½ teaspoon salt	250 g (9 oz) cannellini beans, undrained
½ teaspoon pepper	
pinch of dried chilli flakes	2 tablespoons grated Pecorino (Romano) or Parmesan cheese (optional)

In a large saucepan, heat the oil, garlic, salt, pepper and chilli flakes over medium heat. Do not let the garlic brown. Add the escarole and stir for 2 to 3 minutes. Add the beans with their liquid. Raise the heat to medium–high and heat the beans through for 1 to 2 minutes.

Remove the pan from the heat. Add the cheese, if using.

Makes 4 servings

NUTRITION AT A GLANCE
Per serving: Energy 220 cals/920 kJ; 15 g fat (of which 3 g saturates), 8 g protein, 13 g carbohydrate (of which 2 g sugars), 4 g fibre, 474 mg sodium

Barley with Mushrooms

The meaty and full-flavoured mushrooms combine with the nuttiness from the barley and cheese to make this a true winner.

15 g (½ oz)	dried porcini mushrooms
240 ml (8 fl oz)	hot water
3	tablespoons extra virgin olive oil
4	cloves garlic, finely chopped
170 g (6 oz)	portobello or chestnut mushroom caps, chopped
1	bunch spring onions, finely chopped
850 ml (1½ pints)	vegetable stock
200 g (7 oz)	pearl barley
	salt
	freshly ground black pepper
60 g (2 oz)	Pecorino (Romano) cheese, grated
30 g (1 oz)	Parmesan cheese, grated

Put the porcini mushrooms in a bowl and cover with the hot water. Set aside.

Heat the oil in a large frying pan over medium–high heat. Add the garlic and chopped mushrooms and cook, stirring occasionally, for 10 minutes, or until they begin to brown.

Drain the porcini mushrooms, then cut into small pieces and add to the frying pan. Cook for 1 minute. Add 2 tablespoons of the spring onions, the stock, barley, and salt and pepper to taste. Bring to simmering point. Reduce the heat to low, cover and simmer for 12 minutes, or until almost all of the liquid is absorbed. Remove from the heat and add the Pecorino cheese. Just before serving, add the remaining spring onions and sprinkle with the Parmesan.

Makes 4 servings

NUTRITION AT A GLANCE
Per serving: Energy 384 cals/1607 kJ; 18 g fat (of which 6 g saturates), 13 g protein, 45 g carbohydrate (of which 1 g sugars), 1 g fibre, 563 mg sodium

Garlic and Lemon Grilled Vegetables

Give the vegetables a little time to marinate to soak up extra flavour. If you like, you can prepare them a day or two in advance, then cook them up quickly when you're ready.

4	tablespoons chopped fresh flat-leaved parsley
3–4	tablespoons lemon juice
2	tablespoons extra virgin olive oil
3	cloves garlic, finely chopped
1	teaspoon Italian herb seasoning
½	teaspoon ground black pepper
¼	teaspoon salt
2	large red peppers (capsicums), cut into strips
170 g (6 oz)	portobello or chestnut mushrooms, sliced
1	large red onion, halved and cut into 2-cm (¾-in) thick slices

In a large bowl, combine the parsley, lemon juice, oil, garlic, Italian seasoning, black pepper and salt. Add the red peppers, mushrooms and onion and toss to coat well. Leave to marinate for at least 30 minutes. (The mixture can be prepared ahead to this point and refrigerated for up to 2 days.)

Line a grill pan with foil, add the grill rack and coat with cooking spray, or coat a ridged grilling pan with cooking spray. Preheat the grill or pan to medium–hot.

Grill the vegetables, turning often, for 15 minutes, or until very tender and lightly charred.

Makes 4 (side dish) servings

NUTRITION AT A GLANCE
Per serving: Energy 100 cals/418 kJ; 6 g fat (of which 1 g saturates), 3 g protein, 10 g carbohydrate (of which 7 g sugars), 2.5 g fibre, 201 mg sodium

Baked Mushrooms with Melted Goat's Cheese

For a super lunch or dinner, serve these delicious mushrooms with a fresh green salad.

240 ml (8 fl oz) South Beach Tomato Sauce (see page 156)
or low-sugar pasta sauce

4 large mushroom caps

115 g (4 oz) mild goat's cheese, cut into 4 pieces

2 tablespoons pine nuts, chopped

1 tablespoon chopped fresh basil

sprigs of basil, to garnish

Preheat the oven to 190°C/375°F/gas 5.

Spread the sauce in the bottom of a baking dish just large enough to hold the mushrooms in a single layer. Arrange the mushrooms, gill side up, on top. Place a piece of goat's cheese on each mushroom. Sprinkle evenly with the pine nuts.

Bake for 30 minutes, or until hot and bubbling. Sprinkle with the chopped basil. Garnish with the basil sprigs.

Makes 4 servings

NUTRITION AT A GLANCE
Per serving: Energy 210 cals/879 kJ; 16 g fat (of which 6 g saturates), 9 g protein,
6 g carbohydrate (of which 3 g sugars), 2 g fibre, 623 mg sodium

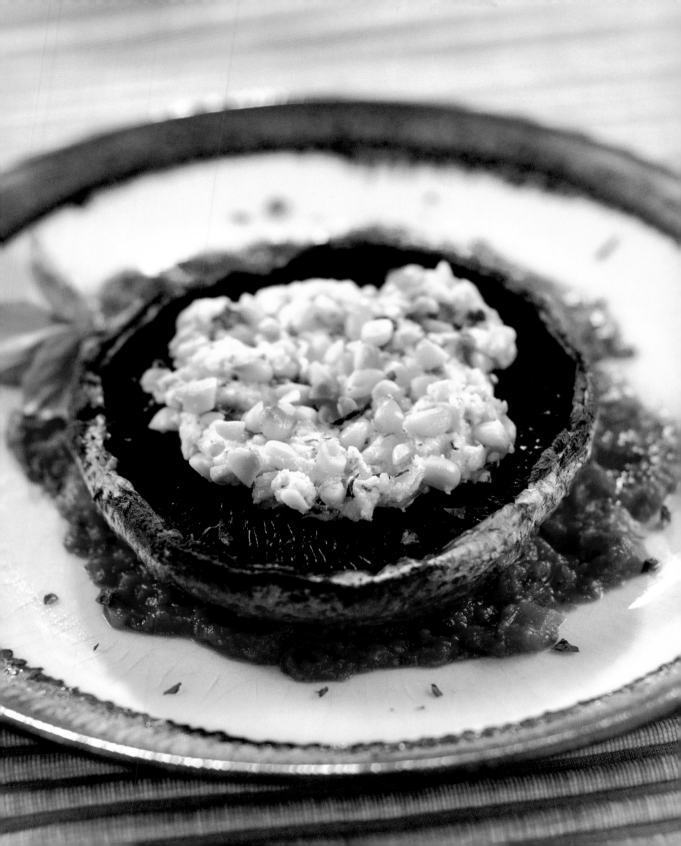

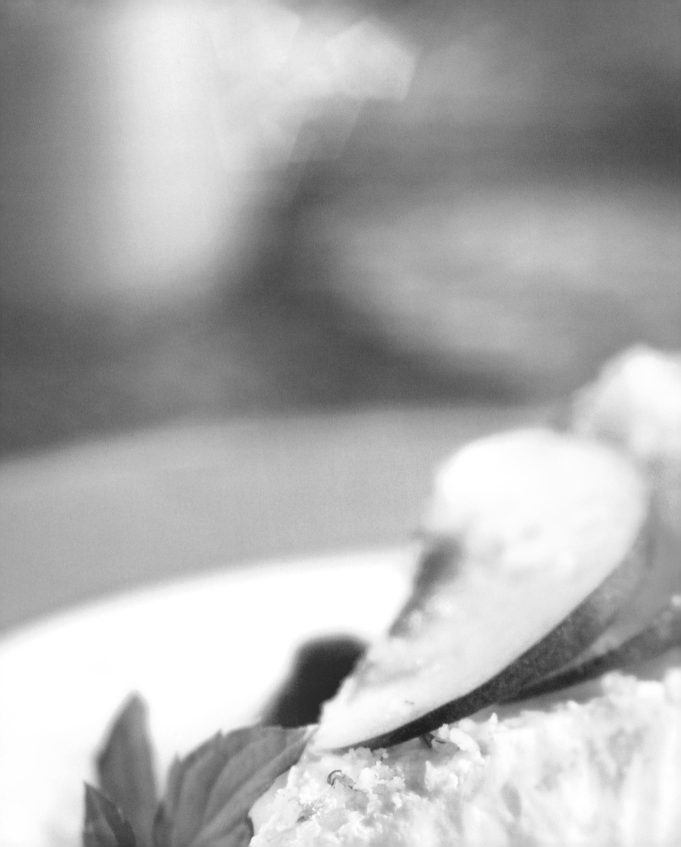

DESSERTS

As I mentioned earlier in this book, I am a chocoholic. That may go some way towards explaining why the South Beach Diet allows you to eat dessert. Our reasoning is simple: a good diet should strive to allow you to eat normally, and for most people, that means having something sweet to round off a meal. We've devised some great desserts that keep to the diet so that you don't have to cheat in order to satisfy your sweet tooth. The truth is, if you use a sugar substitute instead of the real thing, you'll be doing yourself a favour without sacrificing taste. In Phase 1, we suggest low-fat ricotta, fat-free yogurt or fromage frais, which you can sweeten with sugar substitute and flavour with vanilla essence, unsweetened cocoa powder or grated lemon zest. Phase 2 allows fruit and dark chocolate. Steer clear of desserts made from white flour or other processed carbs, and you can indulge on a daily basis and still lose weight.

Chilled Espresso Custard

Complement your meal with coffee at its best — a simply lovely baked custard of rich-tasting espresso.

350 ml (12 fl oz) skimmed milk

2 eggs, beaten

2–3 tablespoons sugar substitute

2 teaspoons espresso powder or instant decaffeinated coffee

1 teaspoon vanilla extract

ground cinnamon, to garnish

In a medium bowl, whisk together the milk, eggs, sugar substitute, coffee and vanilla extract until well blended. Pour into four 180 ml (6 fl oz) custard cups or ramekins and place in a 25 cm (10 in) sauté pan.

Fill the pan with water to 1 cm (½ in) from the tops of the custard cups. Bring the water to the boil over high heat. Reduce the heat to low, cover and simmer for 10 minutes. Remove the cups from the pan, cover with plastic wrap touching the surface of the pudding, and refrigerate for 3 hours, or until chilled. Sprinkle with the cinnamon.

Makes 4 servings

NUTRITION AT A GLANCE
Per serving: Energy 70 cals/293 kJ; 3 g fat (of which 1 g saturates), 6 g protein, 6 g carbohydrate (of which 4 g sugars), 0 g fibre, 83 mg sodium

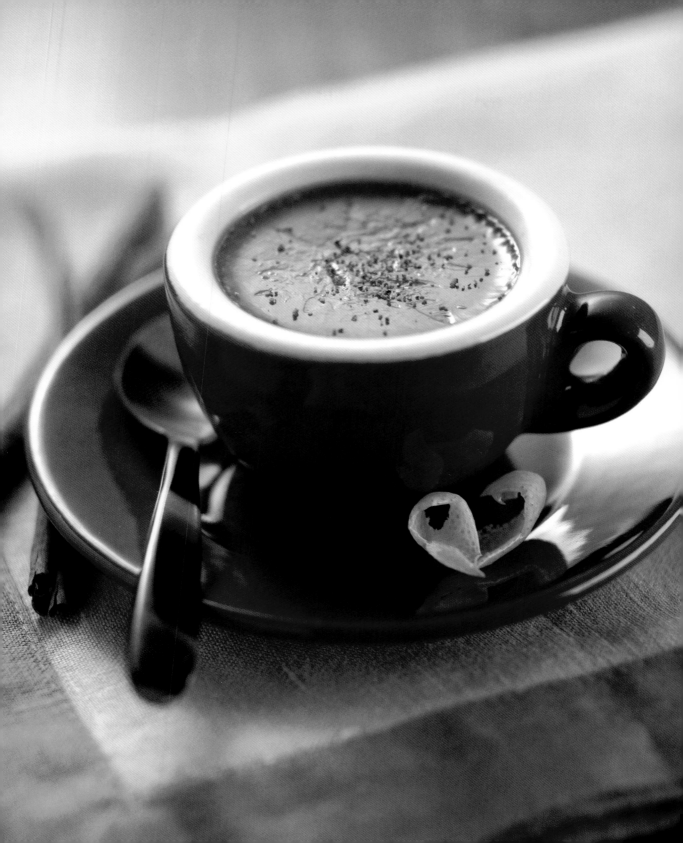

Ricotta Romanoff Sundae

The combination of strawberry and orange flavours is named in honour of the Russian Imperial family. Our version includes ricotta for a satisfying sundae.

250 g (9 oz)	strawberries
½	tablespoon grated orange zest
1½	tablespoons sugar substitute
500 g (1 lb 2 oz)	ricotta cheese (reduced-fat if available)
1	tablespoon pistachios
	mint leaves, to garnish

Cut 145 g (5 oz) of the strawberries into quarters and slice the rest.

In a blender or food processor, combine the quartered strawberries, orange zest and sugar substitute and blend until smooth. Pour into a large bowl. Gently stir in the sliced strawberries. Cover and chill.

When ready to serve, divide the ricotta among 4 serving bowls. Pour equal amounts of the strawberry mixture over the ricotta, then sprinkle with the pistachios. Garnish with the mint leaves.

Makes 4 servings

NUTRITION AT A GLANCE
Per serving: Energy 250 cals/1046 kJ; 16 g fat (of which 10 g saturates), 13 g protein, 8 g carbohydrate (of which 7 g sugars), 1 g fibre, 150 mg sodium

Strawberries with Velvety Chocolate Dip

Strawberries with chocolate dip are so easy to prepare, yet they have an air of luxury. For a special presentation, serve the dip in a clear crystal bowl on a platter circled with the strawberries.

1	tablespoon unsweetened cocoa powder
1	tablespoon boiling water
1	tablespoon sugar substitute
6	tablespoons fat-free natural yogurt
1	teaspoon thawed frozen orange juice concentrate
685 g (1½ lb)	strawberries, hulled

In a measuring jug, dissolve the cocoa in the boiling water. Sweeten to taste with the sugar substitute.

In a small bowl with an electric mixer on medium speed, whip the yogurt, chocolate syrup and orange juice concentrate. Cover and chill until ready to serve. Serve with the strawberries for dipping.

Note: if you can obtain sugar-free chocolate syrup, use 6 tablespoons and whip with the yogurt and orange juice concentrate.

Makes 6 servings

NUTRITION AT A GLANCE
Per serving: Energy 60 cals/251 kJ; 1 g fat (of which 0.5 g saturates), 3 g protein, 9 g carbohydrate (of which 9 g sugars), 2 g fibre, 56 mg sodium

Wonton Cups with Fresh Berries

Wonton wrappers are available in the chilled or frozen food section of most Chinese food shops and some supermarkets.

24	wonton wrappers
2	tablespoons trans-fat-free butter substitute, melted
5	tablespoons sugar-free strawberry jam or no-sugar-added pure fruit spread
230 g (8 oz)	fat-free lemon yogurt, or natural yogurt + 1 teaspoon grated lemon zest
170 g (6 oz)	fresh blackberries, blueberries, or raspberries

Preheat the oven to 180°C/350°F/gas 4.

Using a 12-cup non-stick muffin tin, line each cup with a wonton wrapper. Brush the wonton wrappers with a little of the butter substitute. Place a second wrapper diagonally on top of each of the first ones, so that the points of the wrappers make sides to the cup. Brush the second layer of wrappers with a little butter substitute.

Bake for 8 minutes, or until golden brown. Leave to cool, then remove from the tin.

Divide the jam or fruit spread among the wonton cups.

Place the yogurt and lemon zest, if using, in a bowl and fold in 115 g (4 oz) of the berries. Divide the yogurt mixture among the wonton cups. Top with the remaining berries.

Makes 12 servings

NUTRITION AT A GLANCE

Per serving: Energy 60 cals/251 kJ; 3 g fat (of which 0.5 g saturates), 1.5 g protein, 8 g carbohydrate (of which 7 g sugars), 0.5 g fibre, 50 mg sodium

Cherry Baked Apples

This treat is as simple as it is unusual and delicious.

4	cooking apples
½	teaspoon ground cinnamon
40 g (1¼ oz)	dried cherries or raisins
30 g (1 oz)	walnuts, chopped
240 ml (8 fl oz)	diet sparkling cherry drink

Preheat the oven to 190°C/375°F/gas 5.

Using an apple corer or sharp knife, remove the apple cores from the stem ends without cutting the apples all the way through to the base. Place the apples cored side up in a 23 × 23 cm (9 × 9 in) baking dish.

Sprinkle the apples inside and outside with the cinnamon. Spoon the cherries or raisins and the walnuts into the apples. Drizzle a little cherry drink into each apple. Pour the remaining cherry drink into the baking dish.

Bake for 20 minutes, or until the apples are tender.

Makes 4 servings

NUTRITION AT A GLANCE
Per serving: Energy 118 cals/494 kJ; 5 g fat (of which 0.5 g saturates), 2 g protein, 17 g carbohydrate (of which 16 g sugars), 2 g fibre, 8 mg sodium

Berry Granita

Deliciously refreshing, this is the perfect summer dessert.

120 ml (4 fl oz)	water
4	tablespoons sugar substitute
285 g (10 oz)	frozen blueberries, blackberries or raspberries
	grated zest and juice of 1 lemon
	lemon twists, to garnish

In a small saucepan over medium heat, combine the water and sugar substitute. Bring to the boil. Boil for 2 minutes, then set aside to cool to room temperature.

In a food processor fitted with a metal blade, combine the berries, lemon zest, juice and cooled syrup. Pulse for 2 minutes, or until the blueberries are partially crushed. Pour into a small metal bowl and stir a few times with a fork to break up any large pieces. Cover the bowl with foil and place in the freezer overnight.

Spoon into 6 serving glasses and garnish with a lemon twist.

Makes 6 servings

NUTRITION AT A GLANCE
Per serving: Energy 20 cals/84 kJ; 0 g fat, 0.5 g protein,
4 g carbohydrate (of which 3 g sugars), 1.5 g fibre, 1 mg sodium

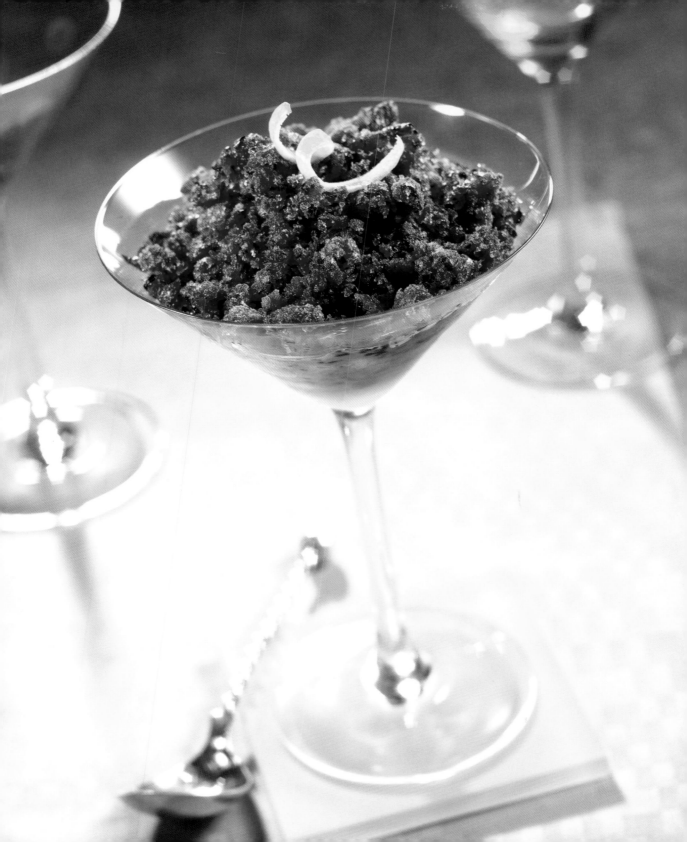

Frozen Strawberry Dessert

Use the berry of your choice, but whatever you do, don't leave this dessert out of your regular repertoire.

2	tablespoons mayonnaise
230 g (8 oz)	reduced-fat cream cheese, softened
1	tablespoon lemon juice
285 g (10 oz)	frozen unsweetened strawberries, partially thawed
2	large egg whites
2	tablespoons sugar substitute

In a medium bowl, blend the mayonnaise and the cream cheese and mix well. Add the lemon juice and strawberries, a little at a time.

Whisk the egg whites until soft peaks form, then add the sugar substitute and whisk until stiff. Fold into the strawberry mixture. Divide the mixture among 6 freezerproof serving dishes and freeze for 2 hours, or until firm.

Makes 6 servings

NUTRITION AT A GLANCE
Per serving: Energy 130 cals/544 kJ; 10 g fat (of which 3 g saturates), 4 g protein, 5 g carbohydrate (of which 5 g sugars), 0.5 g fibre, 80 mg sodium

Strawberry Buttermilk Ice

Is there anyone who doesn't like something smooth and cold on a warm evening?

6	tablespoons sugar substitute
240 ml (8 fl oz)	water
425 g (15 oz)	strawberries, chopped
240 ml (8 fl oz)	buttermilk

In a large bowl, combine the sugar substitute and water. In a blender or food processor, blend the strawberries until smooth. Add the strawberries and buttermilk to the sugar substitute mixture and stir until well combined. Pour into a freezerproof container and freeze overnight.

Remove from the freezer 30 minutes before serving.

Makes 4 servings

NUTRITION AT A GLANCE
Per serving: Energy 65 cals/272 kJ; 0.5 g fat (of which 0 g saturates), 5 g protein, 10 g carbohydrate (of which 10 g sugars), 1.5 g fibre, 26 mg sodium

Strawberry Shimmer

After succeeding with the South Beach Diet, this will be the only thing you see shaking when you walk to the table.

2 sachets (25 g)	sugar-free strawberry-flavoured jelly crystals
240 ml (8 fl oz)	boiling water
250 g (9 oz)	strawberries, crushed with a fork
230 g (8 oz)	fat-free natural yogurt

Coat a 1–litre (1¾–pint) mould with cooking spray.

In a large bowl, dissolve the jelly crystals in the boiling water. Add the strawberries and stir well. Chill for 30 minutes, or until thickened.

Beat with an electric mixer on medium speed until frothy. Fold in the yogurt. Pour the mixture into the prepared mould and chill for 1½ hours, or until firm.

Makes 4 servings

NUTRITION AT A GLANCE
Per serving: Energy 45 cals/188 kJ; 0 g fat, 3 g protein,
8 g carbohydrate (of which 7 g sugars), 1 g fibre, 46 mg sodium

MY SOUTH BEACH DIET

JUST CALL ME 'THE INCREDIBLE SHRINKING GRANNY'.

Two months ago, I weighed in at my doctor's office at 155 kg (24 st) – the heaviest I have ever been. That night I got an e-mail about the South Beach Diet, and I almost deleted it. Luckily, I visited the *Prevention.com* website, and the rest is history.

By the end of Phase 1, I had lost 8 kg (18 lb). In Phase 2, I have been losing about 1.6 kg (3½ lb) a week. I am currently down 16 kg (2½ stone) in only 61 days! I don't exercise yet, but I plan to start once I drop below 136 kg (21 st).

What's great is that almost anything is allowed after the first two weeks. Even in Phase 1, the meals and snacks are plentiful. I was never hungry. I have always cooked lunch and dinner, so it wasn't that hard for me to switch from my regular cooking to South Beach cooking.

Recently, at a birthday party for my 6-year-old granddaughter, I had three bites of a piece of cake. Afterwards, I had a horrible time with cravings for about 24 hours. I wanted chips and cake and biscuits and on and on. Luckily, I was able to fill myself up with South Beach-legal foods, and once I got through that day, I was back on track. That's one way to learn the difference between giving your body the wrong or right fuels.

In the past, I've struggled with chronic health problems like rheumatoid arthritis, chronic fatigue and fibromyalgia. Since starting the South Beach Diet, I have twice as much energy, and my cholesterol level is now well within the normal healthy range. I am able to do so much more with less joint pain. I spend less time resting and more time volunteering at my granddaughter's school. She is so proud that I can be there – a real side benefit I wasn't expecting!

At my recent annual check-up, my doctor said she was impressed enough to go and buy the book and read it for her other patients. She checked my records twice to be sure that the weight recorded two months ago was correct. This is really a way of life, not a quick fix. With my online SB support group, I call myself 'the Incredible Shrinking Granny'. When I'm down to 77 kg (12 st), I'm going to be proud to share who I really am with my granddaughter. I need all the energy and health I can get to keep up with her! – *APRIL G.*

Apple and Almond Soufflé

A very light and fluffy treat for all you dessert lovers out there. Almonds are included for some heart-healthy fat.

3	cooking apples, peeled, cored and cut into bite-size pieces
60 ml (2 fl oz)	water
3	tablespoons sugar substitute
½	teaspoon almond extract
5	egg whites
30 g (1 oz)	sliced almonds, toasted (optional)

Put the apples and water into a 2-litre (4-pint) saucepan. Bring to the boil over high heat. Reduce the heat to low, cover and simmer, stirring occasionally, for 10 minutes, or until the apples are tender. Stir in the sugar substitute and almond extract. Remove from the heat and place the pan in a bowl of ice-cold water for 10 minutes.

Preheat the oven to 220°C/425°F/gas 7.

In a large bowl, using an electric mixer on high speed, beat the egg whites until stiff peaks form. With a rubber spatula, gently fold into the cooled apple mixture. Spoon the mixture into a 1½-litre (2½-pint) soufflé dish.

Bake for 15 minutes, or until the soufflé is puffed and browned. Sprinkle with the almonds, if using. Serve warm.

Makes 4 servings

NUTRITION AT A GLANCE
Per serving: Energy 100 cals/418 kJ; 4 g fat (of which 0.5 g saturates), 6 g protein, 10 g carbohydrate (of which 9 g sugars), 2 g fibre, 79 mg sodium

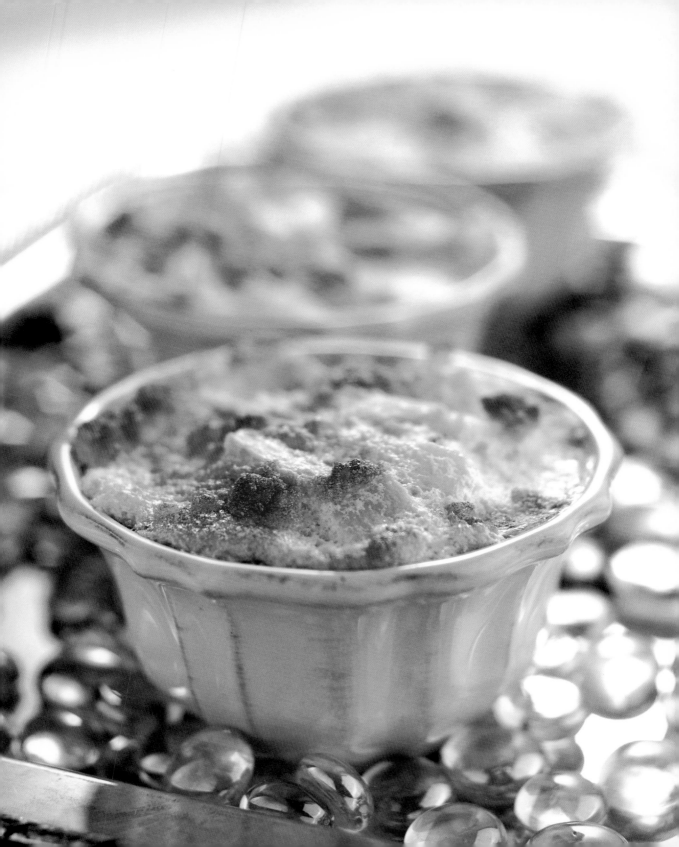

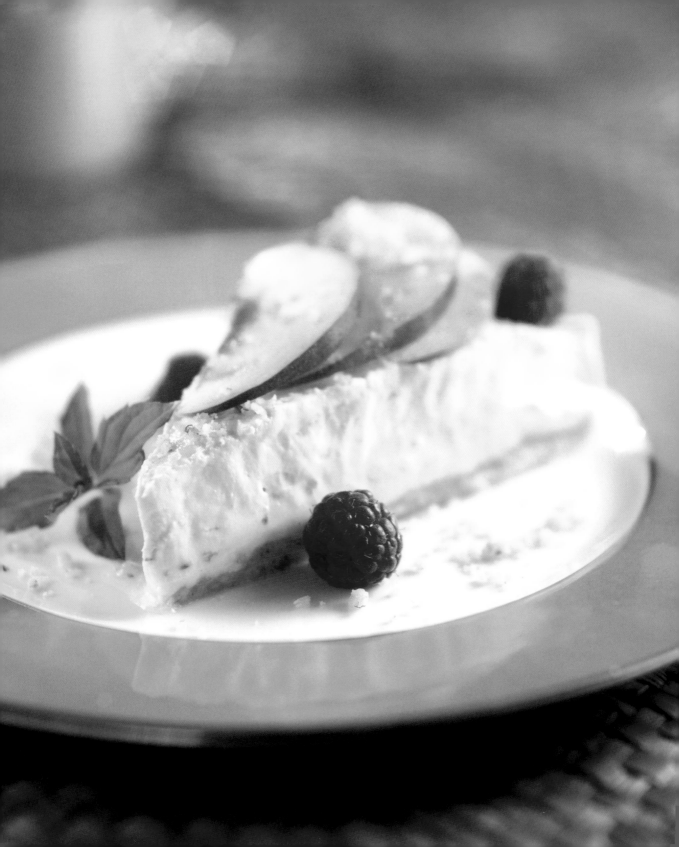

Peachy Walnut Torte

Because the South Beach Diet is ultimately a lifestyle, an occasional indulgence in a little sugar or butter can be allowed. Just savour a small piece. Enjoy!

90 g (3 oz)	walnuts, ground
60 g (2 oz)	trans-fat-free butter substitute or butter
50 g (1¾ oz)	sugar
455 g (1 lb)	reduced-fat cream cheese
6	tablespoons sugar substitute
230 g (8 oz)	fat-free raspberry yogurt
230 g (8 oz)	fat-free peach yogurt
2	drops yellow food colouring (optional)
2–3	large peaches, thinly sliced
	raspberries, to garnish
	sprigs of mint, to garnish

Place one-third of the walnuts in a small bowl and set aside.

Place the remaining walnuts in another small bowl and add the butter substitute (or butter) and sugar. Mix well with a fork. Press the walnut mixture firmly into the bottom of a 20 cm (8 in) diameter springform tin.

In a large bowl, using an electric mixer on medium speed, beat the cream cheese and sugar substitute until smooth. Remove half of the cheese mixture to another bowl and whisk in the raspberry yogurt. Spread evenly over the walnut crust. Place in the freezer for 1 hour, or until firm.

To the remaining cream cheese mixture, add the peach yogurt and food colouring, if using. Cover and refrigerate. When the raspberry layer is firm, spoon the peach mixture over it. Freeze for 2½ hours, or until firm.

When ready to serve, sprinkle with the reserved walnuts, arrange the peach slices on top and decorate with the raspberries and mint.

Makes 10 servings

NUTRITION AT A GLANCE
Per serving: Energy 206 cals/862 kJ; 14 g fat (of which 6 g saturates), 7 g protein, 13 g carbohydrate (of which 13 g sugars), 1 g fibre, 95 mg sodium

Angel Meringue Dessert

This light-as-a-cloud meringue will melt in your mouth.

5	egg whites, at room temperature
⅛	teaspoon salt
¼	teaspoon cream of tartar
30 g (1 oz)	icing sugar, sifted
1½	teaspoons vanilla extract
2	tablespoons finely ground walnuts
250 g (9 oz)	virtually fat-free fromage frais, or 115 g (4 oz) ricotta (reduced-fat if available) + 115 g (4 oz) fat-free natural yogurt
2	tablespoons sugar substitute
115 g (4 oz)	strawberries or raspberries, sliced
	sprigs of mint, to garnish

Preheat the oven to 140°C/275°F/gas 1.

Cover a baking sheet with baking parchment and coat the parchment with cooking spray.

In a large bowl, using an electric mixer on high speed, beat the egg whites and salt until soft peaks form. Gradually sprinkle in the cream of tartar and then the icing sugar, 2 tablespoons at a time, beating well after each addition. Add 1 teaspoon of the vanilla extract and beat until glossy peaks form. Fold in the walnuts. Form the mixture in an 18 cm (7 in) diameter circle on the baking parchment.

Bake for 1 hour, or until light golden. Turn off the oven and let the meringue cool with the door open. Remove from the parchment and store in an airtight container or place on a serving plate.

Using a balloon whisk or fork, whisk the fromage frais (or ricotta and yogurt) with the remaining ½ teaspoon vanilla extract and the sugar substitute. Spread the fromage frais over the meringue, top with the sliced strawberries and garnish with the mint.

Makes 4 servings

NUTRITION AT A GLANCE

Per serving: Energy 150 cals/628 kJ; 7 g fat (of which 1 g saturates), 10 g protein, 14 g carbohydrate (of which 14 g sugars), 1 g fibre, 350 mg sodium

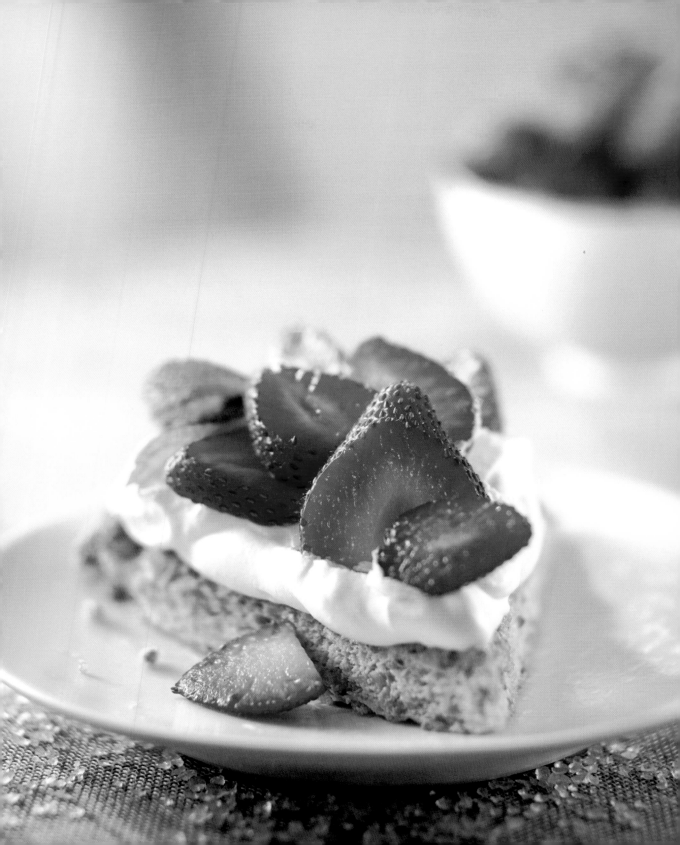

Chocolate Pie with Crispy Peanut Butter Crust

Treat yourself to some chocolate with this easy-to-make pie. The crust, made of toasted-rice cereal, is a crunchy touch that complements the smooth pie.

3	tablespoons unsweetened peanut butter
50 g (1¾ oz)	toasted-rice cereal
1	sachet (50–65 g) no-added-sugar instant chocolate dessert
300 ml (10 fl oz)	skimmed milk

Coat a 20 cm (8 in) or 23 cm (9 in) diameter pie plate with cooking spray.

In a saucepan over low heat, warm the peanut butter until melted. Remove from the heat and stir in the cereal. Press the cereal mixture into the bottom and up the side of the pie plate. Freeze for 1 hour.

Prepare the dessert mix according to the package directions, using the skimmed milk. Pour the mixture into the prepared pie crust. Refrigerate for at least 1 hour before serving.

Makes 8 servings

NUTRITION AT A GLANCE

Per serving: Energy 95 cals/397 kJ; 4.5 g fat (of which 1.5 g saturates), 3.5 g protein, 10 g carbohydrate (of which 4 g sugars), 0.5 g fibre, 160 mg sodium

Chocolate-Swirled Cheesecake

You'll love this South Beach cheesecake, with its tantalizing swirl of chocolate. If you're comfortably into Phase 3, feel free to sprinkle a tablespoon of chocolate chips on top for a crunchy garnish.

60 g (2 oz)	reduced-fat digestive (wheatmeal) biscuits, crushed
750 g (1 lb 10 oz)	ricotta cheese (reduced-fat if available)
4	eggs
90 g (3 oz)	caster sugar
5	tablespoons sugar substitute
80 ml (3 fl oz)	skimmed milk
60 g (2 oz)	plain chocolate, melted

Preheat the oven to 160°C/325°F/gas 3.

Coat a 22 cm (8½ in) diameter springform tin or loose-bottomed cake tin with cooking spray. Sprinkle the bottom of the tin with the biscuit crumbs.

In a large bowl, using an electric mixer on medium speed, beat the cheese until light and fluffy. Add the eggs, sugar, sugar substitute and milk and beat for 4 minutes, or until the mixture is smooth. Pour one-third of the mixture into a small bowl and beat the melted chocolate into it.

Pour the plain mixture into the prepared tin. Top with the chocolate mixture. Using a knife, swirl the mixtures to create a marbled effect. Place the tin in a roasting tin filled with 2 cm (¾ in) water.

Bake for 45 minutes, or until the edges are lightly browned and the centre is nearly set. Cool in the tin on a rack for 30 minutes, then refrigerate overnight.

Makes 12 servings

NUTRITION AT A GLANCE
Per serving: Energy 181 cals/758 kJ; 11 g fat (of which 5 g saturates), 8 g protein, 8 g carbohydrate (of which 6 g sugars), 0 g fibre, 50 mg sodium

Flourless Chocolate Cake with Almonds

It's a rare person who doesn't love chocolate cake! This flourless version looks somewhat flat after baking, but the taste is far from it! Almonds and dark chocolate provide a rich, decadent taste in every bite.

2	tablespoons trans-fat-free butter substitute or unsalted butter
1	tablespoon unsweetened cocoa powder
75 g (2½ oz)	ground almonds
100 g (3½ oz)	caster sugar
90 g (3 oz)	plain chocolate (high cocoa solids)
125 g (4½ oz)	fat-free natural yogurt
4	tablespoons sugar substitute
2	egg yolks
1	teaspoon vanilla extract
¼	teaspoon almond extract (optional)
5	egg whites, at room temperature
¼	teaspoon salt
1	tablespoon toasted slivered almonds (optional)

Preheat the oven to 180°C/350°F/gas 4.

Generously coat a 22 cm (8½ in) diameter springform or loose-bottomed cake tin with 2 teaspoons of the butter substitute and dust with the cocoa powder. (Don't tap out the excess cocoa; leave it in the tin.)

Combine the almonds with 2 tablespoons of the sugar.

In the top of a double boiler over barely simmering water, melt the chocolate and the remaining 4 teaspoons butter, stirring occasionally, until smooth. Remove from the heat. Place the chocolate mixture in a large bowl. Add the almond mixture, yogurt, sugar substitute, egg yolks, vanilla extract, almond extract (if using) and 4 tablespoons of the remaining sugar. Stir until well blended.

In a large bowl, using an electric mixer on high speed, beat the egg whites with the salt until frothy. Gradually add the remaining 2 tablespoons sugar, beating until stiff, glossy peaks form.

Stir one-quarter of the beaten whites into the chocolate mixture to lighten it. Gently fold in the remaining whites until no white streaks remain. Place in the prepared tin. Gently smooth the top.

Bake for 30 to 40 minutes, or until the cake has risen, the top is dry, and a cocktail stick inserted in the centre comes out with a few moist crumbs.

Place the tin on a rack and leave to cool. The cake will fall dramatically. Loosen the edges of the cake with a knife and remove the sides of the tin. Sprinkle with the toasted almonds, if using.

Makes 12 servings

NUTRITION AT A GLANCE
Per serving: Energy 162 cals/678 kJ; 10 g fat (of which 3 g saturates), 5 g protein, 15 g carbohydrate (of which 14 g sugars), 1 g fibre, 131 mg sodium

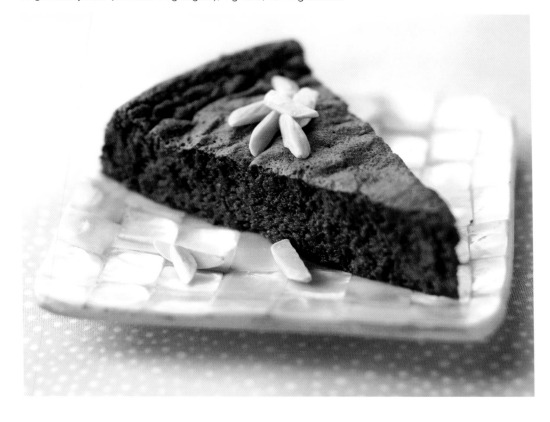

Spice Cake

This is a great alternative to fruit cake or gingerbread for birthdays and celebrations.

185 g (6½ oz)	wholemeal flour
1	teaspoon baking powder
1	teaspoon bicarbonate of soda
1	teaspoon ground nutmeg
1	teaspoon ground cinnamon
½	teaspoon ground allspice
	pinch of salt
90 g (3 oz)	sugar
2–3	tablespoons sugar substitute
2	eggs, beaten
170 g (6 oz)	unsweetened apple sauce
80 ml (3 fl oz)	rapeseed (canola) oil

Preheat the oven to 190°C/375°F/gas 5.

In a large bowl, combine the flour, baking powder, bicarbonate of soda, nutmeg, cinnamon, allspice and salt.

In another large bowl, combine the sugar, sugar substitute, eggs, apple sauce and oil. Pour the egg mixture into the flour mixture and mix thoroughly. Pour into a 23 cm (9 in) diameter cake tin.

Bake for 45 minutes, or until a thin skewer inserted in the centre comes out clean. Cool in the tin on a rack.

Makes 8 servings

NUTRITION AT A GLANCE
Per serving: Energy 230 cals/962 kJ; 11 g fat (of which 1 g saturates), 5 g protein, 30 g carbohydrate (of which 14 g sugars), 2 g fibre, 234 mg sodium

New York-Style Cheesecake

Ah, cheesecake New York-style. It just doesn't get any better! So close your eyes and imagine capping off a delicious al fresco dinner in one of the city's best restaurants with this creamy delight.

1 kg (2¼ lb)	ricotta cheese (reduced-fat if available)
3	eggs, separated
2	tablespoons honey
4	tablespoons sugar substitute
3	tablespoons cornflour
1	tablespoon vanilla extract
30 g (1 oz)	reduced-fat digestive (wheatmeal) biscuits, crushed

Preheat the oven to 180°C/350°F/gas 4.

In a large bowl, beat the cheese until smooth. Stir in the egg yolks, honey, sugar substitute, cornflour and vanilla extract, mixing until thoroughly combined.

In a medium bowl, whip the egg whites until soft peaks form. Fold the whites into the cheese mixture.

Coat a 22 cm (8½ in) diameter springform or loose-bottomed cake tin with cooking spray and cover the bottom of the tin with the biscuit crumbs. Pour the cheese mixture into the tin.

Bake for 30 to 40 minutes, or until golden and set. Cool in the tin on a rack.

Makes 10 servings

NUTRITION AT A GLANCE
Per serving: Energy 187 cals/782 kJ; 9 g fat (of which 5 g saturates), 9 g protein, 18 g carbohydrate (of which 9 g sugars), 0 g fibre, 75 mg sodium

Light as a Feather Lemon Biscuits

These lemony baked treats are an elegant final touch to any meal.

170 g (6 oz)	plain flour
3	tablespoons sugar substitute
3	tablespoons icing sugar
1½	tablespoons grated lemon zest
1	teaspoon baking powder
60 g (2 oz)	trans-fat-free butter substitute, well chilled
1	egg, beaten
1	tablespoon fresh lemon juice
1	tablespoon icing sugar, to dust

In a food processor, combine the flour, sugar substitute, icing sugar, lemon zest and baking powder. Add the butter substitute and pulse on and off until coarse crumbs form. Add the egg and lemon juice and process just until a dough forms.

Form the dough into a ball and wrap it in plastic wrap. Refrigerate the dough for at least 1 hour, or until firm.

Preheat the oven to 180°C/350°F/gas 4. Coat a baking sheet with cooking spray.

Shape the dough into 2.5 cm (1 in) balls and place them 2.5 cm (1 in) apart on the prepared baking sheet.

Bake for 10 minutes, or until the biscuits are golden. Remove the biscuits from the baking sheet and cool on a rack. Dust them with the icing sugar.

Makes 24 biscuits

NUTRITION AT A GLANCE
Per biscuit: Energy 59 cals/247 kJ; 2 g fat (of which 0.5 g saturates), 1 g protein, 9 g carbohydrate (of which 4 g sugars), 0 g fibre, 43 mg sodium

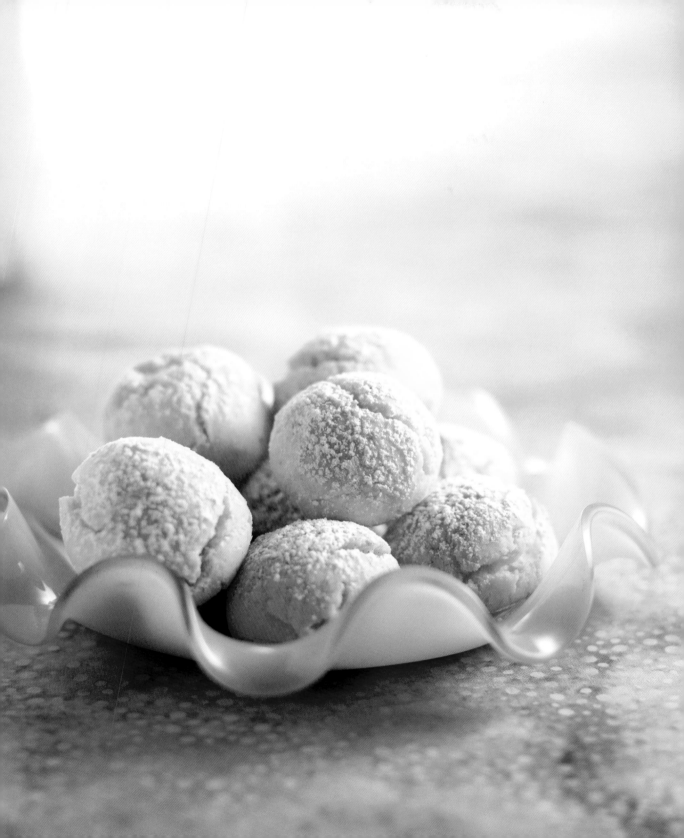

Lemon Cheesecake

Cheesecake was one of man's earliest treats — may the tradition continue.

455 g (1 lb)	ricotta cheese (reduced-fat if available)
455 g (1 lb)	low-fat cottage cheese (1.5% fat or less), fromage frais or quark
5	tablespoons sugar substitute
75 g (2½ oz)	caster sugar
1½	teaspoons cornflour
	juice of 1 lemon
1½	teaspoons plain flour
4	eggs
2	teaspoons vanilla extract
230 g (8 oz)	fat-free natural yogurt

Preheat the oven to 200°C/400°F/gas 6.

Coat a 22 cm (8½ in) diameter springform or loose-bottomed cake tin with cooking spray and line the sides with a double layer of 15-cm (6 in) wide (high) greaseproof paper.

In a large bowl, using an electric mixer on medium speed, blend the ricotta cheese, cottage cheese, 4 tablespoons of the sugar substitute and the sugar until smooth. Beat in the cornflour, lemon juice, flour, eggs and 1 teaspoon of the vanilla extract. Pour the batter into the prepared tin.

Bake for 1 hour and 10 minutes, or until the top of the cake is brown. Turn the oven off and leave the cake in the oven for a further 1 hour.

In a medium bowl, combine the yogurt, the remaining 1 tablespoon sugar substitute and the remaining 1 teaspoon vanilla extract. Spread over the cheesecake and return to the oven for 10 minutes. Refrigerate for 8 hours or overnight before slicing.

Makes 10 servings

NUTRITION AT A GLANCE
Per serving: Energy 148 cals/620 kJ; 3 g fat (of which 1 g saturates), 14 g protein, 17 g carbohydrate (of which 15 g sugars), 0 g fibre, 238 mg sodium

New-Fashioned Peanut Butter Cookies

Old-fashioned cookies with a new-fashioned South Beach twist.

6	tablespoons trans-fat-free butter substitute, softened
115 g (4 oz)	unsweetened smooth peanut butter, at room temperature
4	tablespoons brown sugar substitute or soft brown sugar
4	tablespoons sugar substitute
1	large egg, at room temperature, lightly beaten
1	teaspoon vanilla extract
200 g (7 oz)	oat flour, sifted
¼	teaspoon baking powder
3	tablespoons salted peanuts, chopped

Place an oven rack in the middle position and preheat the oven to 180°C/350°F/gas 4.

In a large bowl, using an electric mixer on medium speed, beat together the butter substitute and peanut butter for 1 minute, or until very smooth. Add the brown sugar and sugar substitutes and beat for 2 minutes, or until well combined and light in colour. Gradually beat in the egg and vanilla extract, beating until very smooth and fluffy. Mix in the flour and baking powder, beating until a moist but cohesive dough forms. Stir in the peanuts.

Drop tablespoonfuls of the mixture about 5 cm (2 in) apart on non-stick baking sheets. Using the tines of a fork dampened in cold water, flatten each in a cross-hatch pattern until 5 cm (2 in) in diameter.

Bake for 15 minutes, or until golden brown. Remove to a rack to cool.

Note: if oat flour is unavailable, make your own: place 200 g (7 oz) + 4 tablespoons rolled oats in a blender or food processor and process until flour-like.

Makes 24 cookies

NUTRITION AT A GLANCE
Per cookie: Energy 120 cals/502 kJ; 8 g fat (of which 1.5 g saturates), 3 g protein, 10 g carbohydrate (of which 4 g sugars), 1 g fibre, 66 mg sodium

CREDITS

The recipe for Artichokes in Olive Oil on page 60 is printed with permission of Antonio Ellek, owner, and Tulin Tuzel and Carla Ellek, chefs, of Pasha's.

The recipe for Casa Tua Tuna Tartare on page 62 is printed with permission of Michele Grendene, owner, and Sergio Sigala, chef, of Casa Tua Restaurant.

The recipe for Wild Mushroom Cappuccino on page 76 is printed with permission of Shareef Malnik, owner, and Andrew Rothschild, chef, of The Forge.

The recipe for Classic Gazpacho with Avocado Crab Farci on pages 86 and 87 is printed with permission of Julian Serrano, executive chef of Picasso.

The recipe for Roasted Yellow Pepper Soup with Broad Beans and Cherry Tomatoes on pages 92 and 93 is printed with permission of Andrea Curto-Randazzo and Frank Randazzo, owners and chefs of Talula Restaurant & Bar.

The recipes for Manhattan Clam Chowder on pages 102 and 103 and Sweet Onion Dressing on page 157 are printed with permission of Jo Ann Bass, owner, and André Bienvenu, chef, of Joe's Stone Crab.

The recipe for Shaved Fennel Salad with Seared Tuna and Parmesan on pages 114 and 115 is printed with permission of the Mandarin Oriental, owner, and Michelle Bernstein, chef, of Azul.

The recipe for Chinese Vegetable Salad with Feta on pages 128 and 129 is printed with permission of Jonathan Eismann, owner and chef of Pacific Time.

The recipe for Grilled Fish on Chopped Salad with Olive Oil Lemon Vinaigrette on pages 170 and 171 is printed with permission of Charlie Hines, managing director, and Marc Ehrler, executive chef, of Preston's at The Loews Miami Beach Hotel.

The recipes for Sea Bass Staten Island Style on pages 174 and 175 and Macaluso's Escarole and Beans on pages 290 and 291 are printed with permission of Michael D'Andrea, owner and chef of Macaluso's.

The recipe for Barbecue Salmon on pages 180 and 181 is printed with permission of Jeffrey Chodorow, owner, and Keyvan Behnam, chef, of China Grill.

The recipe for Shellfish in a Pot on pages 190 and 191 is printed with permission of Barton G. Weiss, owner, and Ted Mendez, chef, of Barton G The Restaurant.

The recipe for Sea Bass with Baby Pak Choi and Soy-Ginger Vinaigrette on pages 194 and 195 is printed with permission of Eric Ripert, owner and chef of Le Bernardin.

The recipes for Asparagus, Crab and Grapefruit Salad on pages 198 and 199 and Grilled Fillet Steak with Roasted Garlic and Chipotle Pepper Chimichurri on pages 252 and 253 are printed with permission of Smith & Wollensky restaurant group and Robert Mignola, chef, of Smith & Wollensky.

The recipe for Spanish Spice-Rubbed Chicken with Mustard and Spring Onion Dressing on pages 208 and 209 is printed with permission of Bobby Flay, owner and chef of Bolo Restaurant & Bar.

The recipe for Japanese Baked Poussin on pages 220 and 221 is printed with permission of Kevin Aoki, owner, and Hiro Terada, chef, of Doraku.

The recipe for Grilled Lamb Loin Salad with Chilled Greek Olive Ratatouille on pages 238 and 239 is printed with permission of Jose Vilarello and Geoffrey Cousineau, chef, of The Biltmore Hotel.

The recipe for Bolivian Spiced Pork Chops on pages 256 and 257 is printed with permission of Norman Van Aken, owner and chef of Norman's.

The recipe for Roasted Pork Tenderloin with Chickpeas, Roasted Peppers and Clams on pages 260 and 261 is printed with permission of Rodrigo Martinez and Tim Andriola, co-owners of Timo.

The recipe for Veal Mignon on pages 264 and 265 is printed with permission of Jeffrey Chodorow, owner, and Claude Troisgros, chef, of Blue Door at Delano.

The recipe for Mediterranean Vegetable Risotto on pages 274 and 275 is printed with permission of Melanie Muss, owner, and Russell Martoccio, chef, of Bleau View at the Fontainebleau Hilton Resort.

The recipe for Caribbean Ratatouille on pages 280 and 281 is printed with permission of Allen Susser, owner and chef of Chef Allen's.

INDEX

Note: Underscored page references indicate boxed text. **Bold** page references indicate photographs.

C

OTHER RODALE BOOKS
AVAILABLE FROM PAN MACMILLAN

1-4050-2101-2	8 Minutes in the Morning	*Jorge Cruise*	£12.99
1-4050-3284-7	Anti-Ageing Prescriptions	*Dr James A. Duke*	£14.99
1-4050-0668-8	Banish Your Belly, Butt and Thighs	*The Editors of* Prevention	£10.99
1-4050-4099-8	Before the Heart Attacks	*Dr H. Robert Superko*	£12.99
1-4050-4179-X	Fit Not Fat at 40+	*The Editors of* Prevention	£12.99
1-4050-7732-8	How to Help Your Overweight Child	*Karen Sullivan*	£12.99
1-4050-3335-5	Picture Perfect Weight Loss	*Dr Howard Shapiro*	£14.99
1-4050-6715-2	South Beach Diet Good Fats/Good Carbs Guide	*Dr Arthur Agatston*	£4.99
1-4050-3340-1	When Your Body Gets The Blues	*Marie-Annette Brown and Jo Robinson*	£10.99

All Pan Macmillan titles can be ordered from our website, *www.panmacmillan.com,* or from your local bookshop and are also available by post from:

Bookpost, PO Box 29, Douglas, Isle of Man IM99 1BQ
Tel: 01624 836000; fax: 01624 670923; e-mail: *bookshop@enterprise.net;*
or visit: *www.bookpost.co.uk.* Credit cards accepted. Free postage and packing in the United Kingdom

Prices shown above were correct at time of going to press.
Pan Macmillan reserve the right to show new retail prices on covers which may differ from those previously advertised in the text or elsewhere.

For information about buying *Rodale* titles in **Australia**, contact Pan Macmillan Australia.
Tel: 1300 135 113; fax: 1300 135 103; e-mail: *customer.service@macmillan.com.au;*
or visit: *www.panmacmillan.com.au*

For information about buying *Rodale* titles in **New Zealand**, contact Macmillan Publishers New Zealand Limited. Tel: (09) 414 0356; fax: (09) 414 0352; e-mail: *lyn@macmillan.co.nz;* or visit: *www.macmillan.co.nz*

For information about buying *Rodale* titles in **South Africa**, contact Pan Macmillan South Africa. Tel: (011) 325 5220; fax: (011) 325 5225; e-mail: *roshni@panmacmillan.co.za*